CASE R

Spine
Imaging

Series Editor
David M. Yousem, MD
Professor, Department of Radiology
Director of Neuroradiology
Johns Hopkins Hospital
Baltimore, Maryland

Other Volumes in the CASE REVIEW Series

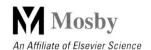

Mosby
An Affiliate of Elsevier Science

Brian C. Bowen, MD, PhD
Associate Professor of Radiology and
Neurological Surgery
Department of Radiology
University of Miami School of Medicine
Miami, Florida

CASE REVIEW

Spine Imaging

CASE REVIEW SERIES

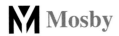

An Affiliate of Elsevier Science

Editor-in-Chief: Richard Lampert
Acquisitions Editor: Stephanie Donley
Manuscript Editor: Amy Norwitz
Production Manager: Peter Faber
Illustration Specialist: John Needles
Book Designer: Gene Harris

Copyright © 2001 by Mosby, Inc.

All rights reserved. No part of this publication may be reproduced or transmitted in any form or by any means, electronic or mechanical, including photocopy, recording, or any information storage and retrieval system, without permission in writing from the publisher.

Permissions may be sought directly from Elsevier's Health Sciences Rights Department in Philadelphia, USA: phone: (+1)215-238-7869, fax: (+1)215-238-2239, email: healthpermissions@elsevier.com. You may also complete your request on-line via the Elsevier Science homepage (http://www.elsevier.com), by selecting 'Customer Support' and then 'Obtaining Permissions'.

Mosby, Inc.
An Affiliate of Elsevier Science
11830 Westline Industrial Drive
St. Louis, Missouri 63146

Printed in United States of America

Library of Congress Cataloging-in-Publication Data

Bowen, Brian C.

Spine imaging: case review / Brian C. Bowen

p.;cm.

ISBN 0–323–00507–1

1. Spine—Imaging.   2. Spine—Diseases—Diagnosis.   I. Title.

[DNLM: 1. Spinal Diseases—radiography—Case Report.   2. Diagnostic
Imaging—methods—Case Report. WE 725 B786s 2001]

RD768 .B656 2001
617.5′60754—dc21

2001030078

Last digit is the print number: 9   8   7   6   5   4   3   2

To Kathryn and Christopher

When I was considering who should write the case review book on spinal imaging to complete the "triptych" for the field of neuroradiology (*Brain Imaging: Case Review* by Laurie A. Loevner and *Head and Neck Imaging: Case Review* by David M. Yousem are already published), I decided to choose a young bright star in the field. Brian Bowen was my choice, and he had the full support of Bob Grossman, the co-author of our *Neuroradiology: THE REQUISITES* textbook. The result of Brian's hard work is a wonderful collection of spine cases that will be useful to all readers of myelograms, MRIs, CTs, spinal arteriograms (conventional and MRAs), and plain films of the spinal canal. Brian's is a very strong contribution to the Case Review series. By reviewing the brain, head and neck, and now the spine books, the reader will gain confidence in his or her interpretations of all neuroradiologic studies.

The Case Review series is designed to review each specialty in a challenging, interactive way. Each book in the series has gradations of difficulty so that the reader can assess his or her proficiency and can use this self-evaluation to guide continued education. By referencing *THE REQUISITES* textbook, the reader can "bone up" on a topic if a weakness is perceived. Because each case in the book is distinct, this text can be picked up and read at any time in your day, or in your career.

I am very pleased to have Dr. Bowen's edition join this very popular, growing series. I welcome *Spine Imaging: Case Review* to the previously published *Obstetric and Gynecologic Ultrasound* by Drs. Johnson and Kurtz; *Musculoskeletal Imaging* by Dr. Yu; *Chest Imaging* by Drs. Boiselle and McLoud; *Genitourinary Radiology* by Drs. Tung, Zagoria, and Mayo-Smith; *Gastrointestinal Radiology* by Drs. Halpert and Feczko; *Brain Imaging* by Dr. Loevner; and *Head and Neck Imaging* by Dr. Yousem. Congratulations to Dr. Bowen on a job well done.

David M. Yousem, MD

Like its predecessors in the neuroradiology portion of the Case Review series, *Head and Neck Imaging* and *Brain Imaging*, this book on imaging of the spine provides case material that illustrates the educational points made in the parent textbook, *Neuroradiology: THE REQUISITES*. In addition, many entities that are discussed only briefly, or not at all, in the textbook are presented and discussed in this casebook. By complementing and supplementing the textbook, my intention has been to reinforce its basic principles and to acquaint the reader with the imaging findings in a wide range of diseases. This wider exposure will hopefully provide an additional measure of confidence to individuals who are preparing for examinations, such as the examinations required for board certification in radiology and for the Certificate of Added Qualification (CAQ) in neuroradiology.

The cases in this book follow the same general format as previous volumes in the Case Review series: questions related to the displayed images, then answers, references, a cross-reference to *THE REQUISITES*, and finally a comment. A description of the findings in each case, however obvious, is included to allow a basis for discussion of the case. For every case, the questions and answers have been drawn from the literature, usually the article(s) referenced in the case. While most of the references are current, some older papers have been referenced because they elucidated the entity being discussed better than subsequent works or because the descriptions of some entities affecting the spine, such as diffuse skeletal hyperostosis, have not significantly changed since earlier published studies. In some cases, a current case report with review of the literature has been used to provide an up-to-date reference as well as a source of previous publications on the topic of interest. In the cases that illustrate a technique or a physical phenomenon, I have attempted to provide an uncomplicated explanation of the entity, accompanied by a reference to a more thorough discussion in the literature.

Brian C. Bowen, MD, PhD

This book would not have been written without the help and support of many people. First, of course, was Dave Yousem, who offered me the opportunity to contribute to the Case Review series, which he has guided and nurtured since its inception. Dave allowed me to review his teaching files, from which 15 of the cases presented here have been drawn. He also allowed me wide latitude in the preparation of the book, and I appreciate his patience during this venture. Managing editor Stephanie Donley brought this work to fruition. From her initial enthusiasm for the first batch of cases to her encouragement during the final stages of the manuscript, Stephanie was attentive to the progress and quality of the work.

I am grateful to my colleagues in diagnostic neuroradiology at the University of Miami—Judy Post, Evelyn Sklar, Steve Falcone, Michelle Whiteman, Alan Holz, and Jane Onufer—for providing an academic milieu in which spinal imaging is emphasized. This milieu is further enriched by our close collaboration with faculty members in the neurological surgery, orthopedic surgery, and neurology departments at UM. Many of these individuals participate in the Miami Project to Cure Paralysis, and several have contributed directly or indirectly to the material in this book. In particular, I wish to thank Alan Holz, Marc Shapiro, and Nathan Lebwohl, each of whom provided several excellent cases. I am also indebted to Vic Haughton of the University of Wisconsin and to Mauricio Castillo and J. Keith Smith of the University of North Carolina for unique case material from their teaching files. The residents in radiology and the fellows in neuroradiology at UM were instrumental in "pilot testing" potential cases, and I am especially grateful to one of the neuroradiology fellows, Efrat Saraf-Lavi, who screened about half the cases and "discovered" some of the most intriguing ones.

I wish to express my sincere appreciation to two individuals in the department of radiology whom I have frequently consulted. Pradip (Fred) Pattany, a talented MR physicist at the UM MR Imaging Center, was the sounding board for my interpretations of the physical phenomena underlying the findings and techniques (including MR angiography, diffusion-weighted imaging, and CSF flow imaging) that are presented in this book. Robert Quencer, chairman of radiology and editor-in-chief of the *American Journal of Neuroradiology*, gave of his valuable time unselfishly, reviewing every case in the book. His comments and suggestions were incisive, and their overall effect, I believe, was to make the text more lucid and consistent from case to case.

Finally, I thank my teenage children, Christopher and Kathryn, who provided plenty of healthy distractions from the writing process and who had the opportunity to see firsthand the demands and the rewards of scholarship.

Brian C. Bowen, MD, PhD

Opening Round

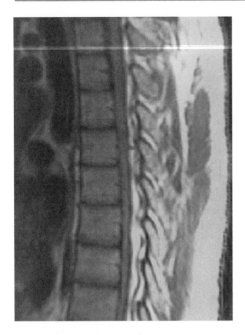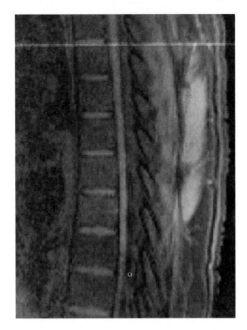

1. In this 33-year-old man with acute exacerbation of progressive myelopathy, what is the diagnosis, based on these two images?

2. Name three causes of this condition.

3. Is this condition more likely to involve the cervical, thoracic, or lumbar spine?

4. What treatment would you consider for this patient?

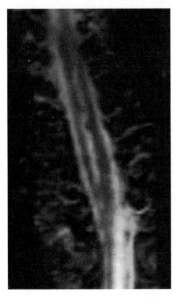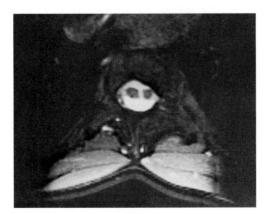

1. Name at least three abnormalities detectable on plain radiographs that are associated with the entity shown above.

2. What structure may be detected within the split spinal cord? Is it always present?

3. At the level of the cleft, how many dorsal and ventral roots are likely to be found?

4. Where is the cleft most likely to occur?

C A S E 1

Epidural Lipomatosis

1. Epidural lipomatosis with thoracic cord compression.

2. The three broad categories are exogenous steroid administration (e.g., in transplant patients and patients treated for chronic medical conditions such as rheumatoid arthritis), elevated endogenous steroid levels (e.g., with adrenal tumors and endocrinopathies), and idiopathic epidural lipomatosis (almost exclusively in the obese population).

3. Approximately equal involvement of the thoracic spine and lumbar spine. Cervical spine involvement is extremely rare.

4. Decompressive laminectomy is recommended for patients with myelopathy or a rapidly progressive neurologic deficit.

References

Hierholzer J, Benndorf G, Lehmann T, et al: Epidural lipomatosis: Case report and literature review. *Neuroradiology* 38:343–348, 1996.

Robertson SC, Traynelis VC, Follett KA, Menezes AH: Idiopathic spinal epidural lipomatosis. *Neurosurgery* 41:68–75, 1997.

Cross-Reference

Neuroradiology: THE REQUISITES, p 495.

Comment

MR imaging is the diagnostic test of choice for this condition. The presence of abundant epidural fat causing cord or cauda equina compression is suggested by the characteristic finding of high signal intensity on T1-weighted images, which is suppressed with fat saturation techniques (as shown in the second figure), and by intermediate signal intensity on T2-weighted images. Spinal epidural lipomatosis is a rare condition. Patients usually have signs and symptoms of Cushing's syndrome and are predominantly male ($\geq$75%). Lipomatosis consists of unencapsulated, diffuse fatty tissue derived from preexisting epidural fat by hypertrophy, whereas lipomas or angiolipomas are well encapsulated and circumscribed. Management depends on the clinical findings. For patients with cord compression and (rapidly) progressive myelopathy, emergency decompressive laminectomy is appropriate. For patients who are receiving exogenous steroids and have mild symptoms, reduction or discontinuation of steroid therapy is often an efficacious treatment. This approach is not applicable to patients with acute cord compression, who routinely receive short-term, high-dose steroids to lessen cord injury.

Notes

C A S E 2

Diastematomyelia, Single Dural Sac

1. Spina bifida, widened interpediculate distance, hemivertebra, butterfly vertebra, and scoliosis.

2. A fibrous or osteocartilaginous spur or septum. No.

3. The normal segmental complement of two dorsal roots and two ventral roots would be expected at the level of the cleft.

4. The cleft is located below T8 in 85% of cases. In 60% of cases, it involves the lumbar spine only.

Reference

Schlesinger AE, Naidich TP, Quencer RQ: Concurrent hydromyelia and diastematomyelia. *AJNR Am J Neuroradiol* 7:473–477, 1986.

Cross-Reference

Neuroradiology: THE REQUISITES, pp 274–275.

Comment

In diastematomyelia, spinal cord anatomy may range from a partial ventral or dorsal cleft to nearly complete duplication of the cord. Usually, the gray matter of each hemicord forms a dorsal and a ventral horn, giving rise to an ipsilateral segmental dorsal root and a ventral root, respectively. True duplication of the cord, with two sets of dorsal and ventral roots, is called diplomyelia and is rare. Vertebral anomalies, the most common of which are listed in answer 1, are present in 85% of cases. An anterior-posterior spur or septum extending through the canal at the level of the cleft is seen in a variable percentage of patients and is not necessary for the definition of diastematomyelia.

Notes

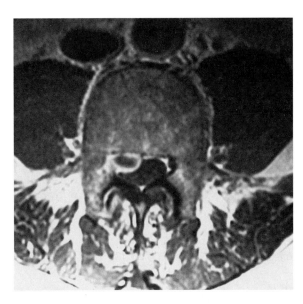
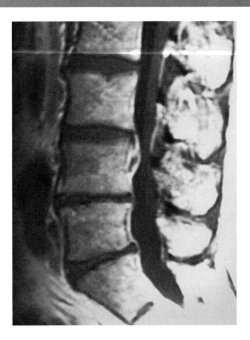

1. Name three lesions that may produce the enhancement pattern shown on the postcontrast T1-weighted axial image from a nonoperated patient.

2. How does the sagittal image help narrow this differential diagnosis?

3. Which nerve root is affected by the lesion?

4. What is enhancing?

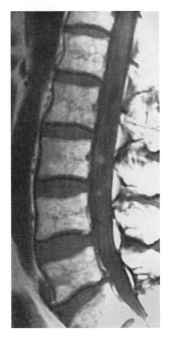
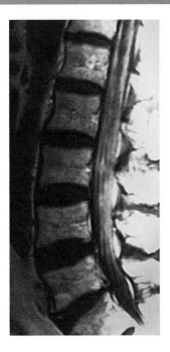

1. What are the most common causes of intradural (leptomeningeal) metastases?

2. Where along the spinal axis are they most likely to be found?

3. Postcontrast spinal MR imaging detects leptomeningeal metastases in what percentage of patients who have positive initial CSF cytology? Negative initial CSF cytology?

4. Which nonmalignant conditions may mimic leptomeningeal metastases?

C A S E 3

Disk Herniation (Sequestration), Lumbar

1. Sequestered disk, epidural abscess, or less likely, schwannoma with cystic degeneration.

2. The enhancement extends to the periphery of the L3-4 disk space, where the linear pattern of enhancement suggests an anular tear and herniated disk.

3. Right L4 root.

4. Vascular fibrous tissue, also called granulation tissue, surrounding the free disk fragment is enhancing.

Reference

Akansel G, Haughton VM, Papke RA, Censky S: Diffusion into human intervertebral disks studied with MR and gadoteridol. *AJNR Am J Neuroradiol* 18:443-445, 1997.

Cross-Reference

Neuroradiology: THE REQUISITES, pp 461-463.

Comment

A sequestered disk, or free fragment, is a portion of herniated disk material that perforates the anulus fibrosus and is not in continuity with the parent disk. The fragment is usually isointense relative to the parent disk on T1-weighted images and isointense to hyperintense on T2-weighted images, presumably because hydration of the fragment is maintained. Thus, the signal characteristics may mimic those of extradural or intradural extramedullary tumors such as schwannoma, neurofibroma, or meningioma. The peripheral enhancement pattern, as shown in this example, helps differentiate a free fragment from these tumors; however, careful technique and interpretation are advised because disk material may be enhanced on delayed scans. Fat saturation pulse sequences help distinguish enhancing granulation tissue from epidural fat on postcontrast images.

Notes

C A S E 4

Leptomeningeal Metastases (Melanoma)*

1. Breast and lung primary carcinomas, melanoma, and non-Hodgkin's lymphoma.

2. Cauda equina.

3. Approximately 90% and 60%, respectively.

4. Granulomatous disease, arachnoiditis, and neurofibromatosis.

References

Gomori JM, Heching N, Siegal T: Leptomeningeal metastases: Evaluation by gadolinium enhanced spinal magnetic resonance imaging. *J Neurooncol* 36:55-60, 1998.

Holtz AJ: The sugarcoating sign. *Radiology* 208:143-144, 1998.

Cross-Reference

Neuroradiology: THE REQUISITES, pp 487-489.

Comment

Diffuse leptomeningeal metastatic disease, or "carcinomatosis," has become more common as the longevity of patients with cancer has increased and as techniques for the identification of malignant cells in CSF have improved. Cauda equina metastases may result from hematogenous spread or intrathecal CSF spread (drop metastases) of malignant cells. The primary CNS neoplasms that have a propensity for drop metastases are glioblastoma multiforme, medulloblastoma, ependymoma, and choroid plexus carcinoma. On postcontrast T1-weighted images, leptomeningeal carcinomatosis may appear as diffuse linear and nodular areas of enhancement along the surface of the spinal cord and cauda equina. This manifestation has been called the "sugarcoating" or "frosting" sign.

---

*Figures for Case 4 from Holtz AJ: The sugarcoating sign. *Radiology* 208:143-144, 1998.

Notes

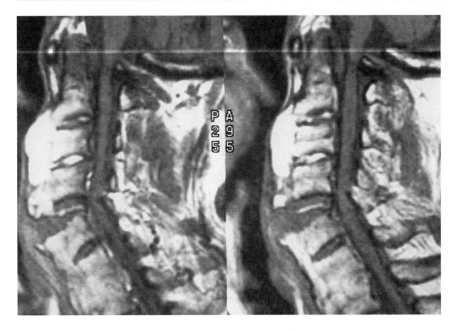

1. How would you classify this injury with regard to mechanism? Is it atypical?
2. Is this patient likely to be HLA-B27 seropositive?
3. Is fusion of the facet joints a manifestation of this disorder?
4. Are patients with this disorder at increased risk for spinal canal stenosis?

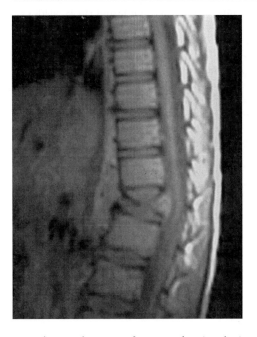
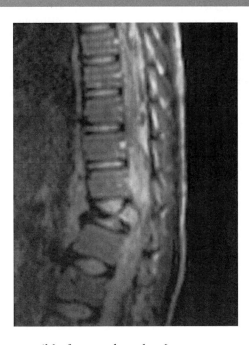

1. What is the most frequent benign lesion responsible for vertebra plana?
2. What are the two most common skeletal locations for this lesion?
3. Among malignant tumors, which most frequently cause vertebra plana?
4. Which of the osseous dysplasias produce vertebral changes that may simulate vertebra plana?

CASE 7

Multilevel Diskitis/Osteomyelitis*

1. In initial studies by Modic and colleagues in 1985, vertebral osteomyelitis was detected with a sensitivity of 96%, a specificity of 92%, and an accuracy of 94%. The sensitivity is probably greater now given the improvements in MR imaging equipment and techniques.

2. The involvement of several vertebral bodies and a prevertebral enhancing mass, suggesting spread along the anterior longitudinal ligament, favor a diagnosis of tuberculous spondylitis.

3. This practice has been controversial because of the high sensitivity and specificity of noncontrast MR imaging; however, gadolinium enhancement can be helpful (see Comment).

4. Yes. In two thirds of cases, infection involves a single disk space and the adjacent vertebral bodies.

References

Post MJD, Bowen BC, Sze G: Magnetic resonance imaging of spinal infection. *Rheum Dis Clin North Am* 17:773-794, 1991.

Modic MT, Feiglin DH, Piraino DW, Boumphrey F, Weinstein MA, Duchesneau PM, Rehm S: Vertebral osteomyelitis: assessment using MR. Radiology 157:157-166, 1985.

Cross-Reference

Neuroradiology: THE REQUISITES, pp 477-478.

Comment

The characteristic findings of diskitis and osteomyelitis on noncontrast MR imaging are (1) irregularity and destruction of the vertebral body end-plates with interruption of the normal signal void of the cortical end-plates; (2) high signal intensity in the disk on T2-weighted images, usually associated with loss of the normal low–signal intensity intranuclear cleft in adults; (3) alteration in height of the disk space; (4) high signal intensity on T2-weighted images and low signal intensity on T1-weighted images within adjacent vertebral bodies; and (5) soft tissue changes around the spine, usually of inhomogeneous signal on both T1- and T2-weighted images. Gadolinium enhancement has proved useful in cases in which the disk space findings are equivocal or the extent of paraspinal or epidural soft tissue changes is poorly shown. For example, in a patient with clinically suspected spinal infection, a disk space narrowed by previous trauma or degenerative disease can yield equivocal findings on noncontrast MR imaging; however, gadolinium enhancement of the disk favors the presence of infection. In patients with epidural or paraspinal abscess, enhancement of the abscess allows more accurate determination of the extent of the mass. Peripheral enhancement of epidural abscess, as shown here at the T8 level, has been observed less often than homogeneous enhancement. Gadolinium enhancement can demonstrate the continuity between an infected disk space and a paraspinal mass, which may be biopsied more easily for diagnosis.

*Figures for Case 7 from Madsen PW III, Bowen BC: Spinal cord disease. In: Kelley RE, Ed: *Functional Neuroimaging.* Armonk, NY, Futura, 1994.

Notes

CASE 8

Intradural Meningioma, Thoracic

1. Extramedullary intradural.

2. Schwannoma.

3. Schwannoma, meningioma, and lipoma.

4. The age and sex of the patient and whether the patient has a history of neurofibromatosis.

Reference

Quekel LGBA, Versteege CWM: "Dural tail sign" in MRI of spinal meningiomas. *J Comput Assist Tomogr* 19:890-892, 1995.

Cross-Reference

Neuroradiology: THE REQUISITES, p 489.

Comment

Intraspinal meningiomas, which represent 25% of intraspinal tumors, occur predominantly in women (F/M = 4:1) and usually in the thoracic spine. The peak age is 45 years. Patients with neurofibromatosis type 2 have a high incidence of schwannomas, meningiomas, and ependymomas. Because meningiomas have a dural base, approximately 85% project intradurally; the remainder are either extradural or both intradural and extradural in location. Psammomatous calcification is commonly present microscopically, yet gross calcification that can be detected on imaging studies, such as CT, is uncommon (<5% of cases). Meningiomas are usually isointense to gray matter but may be lower in signal intensity, depending on the extent of calcification. They are well circumscribed and often show homogeneous enhancement. A "dural tail" may be present, although this finding is nonspecific and may be seen in cases of leptomeningeal metastasis, sarcoidosis, lymphoma, and chloroma. An axial or coronal image is important to show the cord displacement and widening of the subarachnoid space that characterize an extramedullary intradural lesion. Other lesions in the differential diagnosis include schwannoma, which is much more likely than meningioma to widen a neural foramen, and leptomeningeal metastases, which are more likely to be multiple or show diffuse linear enhancement in addition to nodular enhancement.

Notes

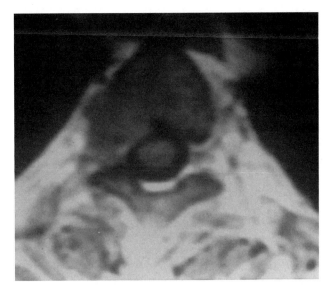
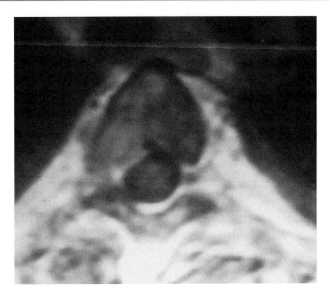

1. What is the most frequent site of metastatic disease to the spine?

2. Which metastases are associated with osteoblastic changes?

3. What findings on T1- and T2-weighted images suggest pathologic fracture rather than osteoporotic vertebral collapse?

4. Why are fast-spin-echo (FSE) T2-weighted images usually unsatisfactory for the detection of vertebral metastases?

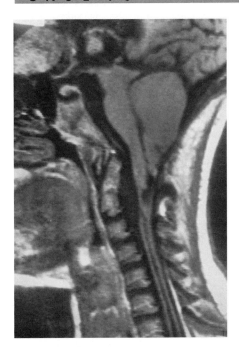

1. Are the abnormal findings on this T1-weighted image caused by a congenital or an acquired disorder?

2. Are the signal changes in the cord best described as hydromyelia, syringomyelia, or myelomalacia?

3. Through what anatomic structure does CSF pass when it travels from the fourth ventricle to the central canal of the spinal cord?

4. Is cervical syrinx more often associated with a Chiari I or Chiari II malformation?

C A S E 9

Vertebral Metastasis (Colon Carcinoma) With Epidural Extension

1. Vertebral body, with subsequent spread to the pedicle and posterior elements.

2. Prostate, breast, ovarian, and transitional cell carcinomas, as well as carcinoid tumor.

3. Diffuse replacement of the entire vertebral body, cortical destruction, involvement of the pedicles and posterior elements, and paraspinal soft tissue abnormalities.

4. Both normal vertebral marrow and tumor-replaced marrow may give hyperintense signal on FSE T2-weighted images. Hyperintensity, caused by fatty marrow, can be suppressed by chemical shift fat saturation or STIR (short tau inversion recovery) techniques.

Reference

Moulopoulos LA, Yoshimitsu K, Johnston DA, Leeds NE, Libshitz HI: MR prediction of benign and malignant vertebral compression fractures. *J Magn Reson Imaging* 6:667–674, 1996.

Cross-Reference

Neuroradiology: THE REQUISITES, pp 491–493.

Comment

Because of its high vascularity, bone marrow in the vertebral body is the most common site for spinal metastases. Initially, fatty marrow is replaced with nonfatty tumor cells. The effect of this change on T1-weighted images, however, depends on the baseline signal intensity of the uninvolved vertebra and on the relative signal intensity of the metastatic lesion. Usually tumor is of lower intensity than marrow, and the metastatic lesion appears hypointense when compared with the uninvolved portion of the vertebra or an adjacent normal vertebra. As shown in this example, however, the metastatic lesion may be isointense relative to the rest of the vertebral body on a T1-weighted image. While other signs suggest tumor, such as involvement of the pedicle and the focal cortical breakthrough shown here, additional evidence is obtained by administering intravenous contrast. On the postcontrast T1-weighted image, tumor within the vertebral body enhances. This finding is almost universal for vertebral metastases, yet it is not pathognomonic because benign vertebral compression fractures may show enhancement. Subtle enhancement of the posterior elements favors a diagnosis of metastasis.

Contrast enhancement also provides better delineation of the extent of epidural invasion, which in this case involves the anterior aspect of the canal and the right neural foramen. The contrast difference between epidural fat and enhancing tumor is further accentuated if fat suppression pulse sequences are used.

Notes

C A S E 1 0

Chiari II Malformation With Hydromyelia

1. Congenital, based on the findings described below.

2. Hydromyelia; however, because we cannot determine on imaging studies whether the cystic cavity is lined by ependymal cells (dilated central canal) or by glial cells (acquired syrinx), the cavity is often referred to as syringohydromyelia.

3. The obex. It is the point on the midline of the dorsal surface of the medulla that marks the narrow, lower portion of the fourth ventricle.

4. Chiari I.

Reference

Samuelsson L, Bergstrom K, Thuomas K-A, et al: MR imaging of syringomyelia and Chiari malformation in myelomeningocele patients with scoliosis. *AJNR Am J Neuroradiol* 8:539–546, 1987.

Cross-Reference

Neuroradiology: THE REQUISITES, pp 261–262.

Comment

The Chiari II malformation is associated with several infratentorial imaging abnormalities, approximately half of which are shown on this T1-weighted sagittal MR image: (1) small posterior fossa; (2) tonsils and medulla herniated through the foramen magnum; (3) fourth ventricle compressed, elongated, and low; (4) beaking of the tectum; (5) enlarged foramen magnum; and (6) low torcular Herophili. In addition to these features, an associated lumbosacral meningocele or meningomyelocele that tethers the cord is nearly always present. Syringohydromyelia, or more specifically, hydromyelia, which represents dilatation of the central canal, may be observed at any cord level but is usually seen in the lower thoracic or lumbar region. In one series of 30 patients (aged 3 to 32 years) with Chiari II malformation and meningomyelocele, 40% had hydromyelia. In Chiari I malformation, hydromyelia is usually cervical in location. For both Chiari I and II, abnormal CSF flow at the foramen magnum is believed to contribute to the pathogenesis of hydromyelia. The cyst-like, dilated central canal communicates with the fourth ventricle via the obex and has CSF-equivalent signal intensity.

Notes

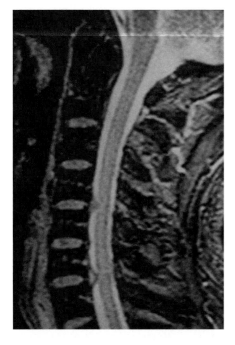
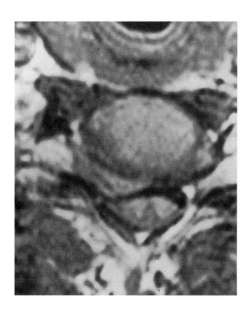

1. Based on the T2*-weighted, gradient-recalled-echo (GRE) sagittal image and the T1-weighted axial image (C6-7 level), did this patient have radiculopathy or myelopathy?

2. Is cervical disk herniation more or less common than lumbar disk herniation?

3. Name one advantage and one disadvantage of fast-spin-echo (FSE) T2-weighted images versus GRE T2*-weighted images.

4. Does the epidural space in the cervical spine contain predominantly fat or venous plexus?

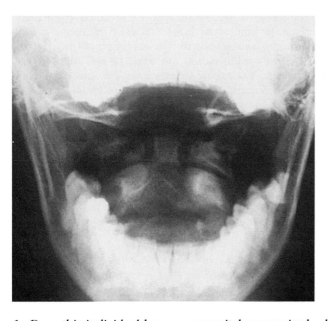
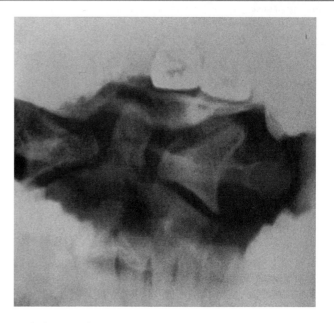

1. Does this individual have a congenital or acquired odontoid abnormality?

2. What imaging study would you recommend next?

3. What is the least common type (Anderson-D'Alonzo classification) of odontoid fracture?

4. What treatment would you recommend for this patient?

Disk Herniation, Cervical*

1. C7 radiculopathy.

2. Less common, in part because the uncinate processes reinforce the disk against posterolateral herniations.

3. FSE T2-weighted scans are less sensitive to susceptibility effects, and therefore spinal osteophytes are not as exaggerated, for example, on sagittal images (which are used to assess central spinal canal narrowing). FSE images, however, are more sensitive to CSF motion artifacts than flow-compensated GRE images are, particularly in the axial plane. FSE T2-weighted images also have less contrast between intervertegbral disk and bone.

4. Venous plexus.

References

Ross JS, Ruggieri PM, Tkach JA, et al: Gd-DTPA–enhanced 3D MR imaging of cervical degenerative disk disease: Initial experience. *AJNR Am J Neuroradiol* 13:127-136, 1992.

Yousem DM, Atlas SW, Hackney DB: Cervical spine disk herniation: Comparison of CT and 3DFT gradient echo MR scans. *J Comput Assist Tomogr* 16:345-351, 1992.

Cross-Reference

Neuroradiology: THE REQUISITES, pp 454, 461-463.

Comment

Spinal lesions that compress and irritate nerve roots cause radiculopathy, whereas lesions that compress the cord produce myelopathy. The midsagittal image in this case shows disk herniations at C4-5 and C6-7; however, no cord compression is present. The C6-7 herniation has a classic "mushroom cap" shape contiguous with the posterior margin of the intervertebral disk space and bordered posteriorly by a thin dark line representing the posterior longitudinal ligament and dura—hence the term *subligamentous herniated disk*. The axial image shows that the herniation is actually posterior-lateral in location. The lateral component protrudes into the right neural foramen and is displacing or compressing the fat and vascular tissue that accompany the C7 nerve root sheath; these changes result in loss of signal intensity in comparison to the normal left neural foramen. Thus, axial views are necessary for the correct diagnosis of cervical disk disease. Axial T2*-weighted images are generally considered more accurate in detecting herniated disks than T1-weighted images are, however, because the T2* weighted images usually have high contrast and often a think dark line between the intermediat- to low-signal herniation and high signal CSF.

---

*Figures for Case 11 from Madsen PW III, Bowen BC: Spinal cord disease. In: Kelley RE, Ed: *Functional Neuroimaging*. Armonk, NY, Futura, 1994.

Notes

Odontoid Fracture, Type II

1. The time interval between the two open-mouth radiographs is 3 years. The right image demonstrates an acute transverse fracture through the junction of the dens and the body of C2.

2. Depends on the clinical picture. In the absence of neurologic symptoms or signs, a helical CT with reformatted sagittal images would be satisfactory for management. In the presence of symptoms, MR images should be obtained to determine whether cervical cord injury or epidural hematoma has occurred.

3. Type I.

4. Because of the high rate of nonunion for type II fractures and potential for atlantoaxial subluxation, C1-C2 (or occiput-C1-C2) fusion is frequently recommended.

References

Anderson LD, D'Alonzo RT: Fractures of the odontoid process of the axis. *J Bone Joint Surg Am* 56:1663-1674, 1974.

Coyne TJ, Fehlings MG, Wallace MC, Bernstein M, Tator CH: C1-C2 posterior cervical fusion: Long-term evaluation of results and efficacy. *Neurosurgery* 37:688-692, 1995.

Dickman CA, Sonntag VK: Posterior C1-C2 transarticular screw fixation for atlantoaxial arthrodesis. *Neurosurgery* 43:275-280, 1998.

Cross-Reference

Neuroradiology: THE REQUISITES, p 501.

Comment

The Anderson-D'Alonzo classification of odontoid fractures recognizes three types: type I is an oblique fracture through the upper portion of the odontoid, type II is a transverse fracture through the base of the odontoid, and type III is a fracture through the body of the axis. The importance of the classification is that type II fractures, which are the most common, may be unstable, whereas type III fractures are usually stable and heal with conservative treatment. A persistent synchondrotic line at the odontoid base may occasionally mimic a type II fracture; however, this line is usually smoother than a true fracture line on plain radiographs. Atlantoaxial subluxation may occur with or without odontoid displacement. In either case, there is a danger of cord compression, which is optimally evaluated with MR imaging. Treatment of atlantoaxial instability is usually posterior C1-C2 wiring with autologous bone grafts. Recently, a higher rate of C1-C2 fusion has been obtained by supplementing this procedure with C1-C2 transarticular screw fixation.

Notes

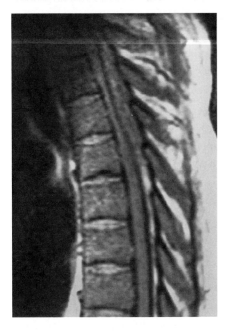 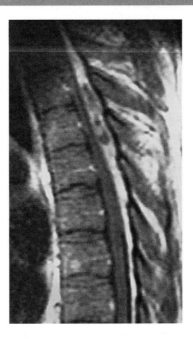

1. Is the lesion shown on the precontrast and postcontrast T1-weighted images of a patient with AIDS more likely to be intradural or extradural? Why?

2. What noninfectious etiology should be considered?

3. Name four factors that are associated with an infectious etiology.

4. If infection is the cause, what is the most likely organism?

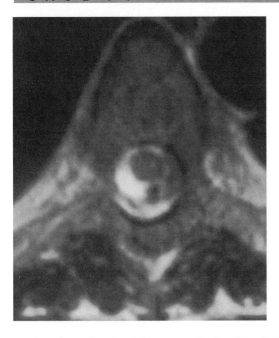 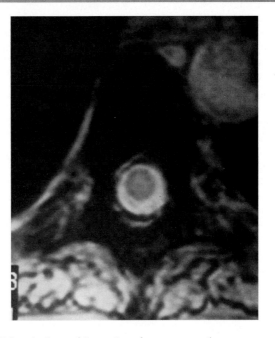

1. Based on these axial images obtained at the T7 level, does this patient have a vascular tumor, vascular malformation, or other lesion?

2. Would another MR technique clarify the findings?

3. What normal structures in the dorsal part of the canal may affect CSF signal intensity?

4. In gradient-echo imaging with a short recovery time (TR) (≤50 msec), what effect best explains the difference in CSF signal intensity on high–flip angle images versus low–flip angle images?

CASE 13

Epidural Abscess, Thoracic

1. Extradural, because on the precontrast image the normal hyperintensity attributable to intact dorsal extradural fat is replaced by the isointense soft tissue mass.

2. Non-Hodgkin's lymphoma.

3. Intravenous drug abuse, diabetes mellitus, previous back trauma, and previous surgery.

4. *Staphylococcus aureus*, whether or not the patient is HIV positive.

Reference

Rigamonti D, Liem L, Sampath P, et al: Spinal epidural abscess: Contemporary trends in etiology, evaluation, and management. *Surg Neurol* 52:189–196, 1999.

Cross-Reference

Neuroradiology: THE REQUISITES, p 479.

Comment

In the precontrast image the normal dorsal epidural fat signal is absent in the upper half of the figure. This same region demonstrates peripheral enhancement with cephalic and caudal areas of more homogeneous enhancement. The mass is compressing the cord. The vertebral bodies appear relatively hypointense when compared with the intervertebral disk spaces on the precontrast images. There is no evidence of vertebral osteomyelitis/diskitis or of abnormal cord enhancement. The patient, a 44-year-old man with a history of intravenous drug abuse, complained of fever, back pain, bilateral lower extremity weakness, and urinary incontinence progressing over a period of 8 days.

While *S. aureus* is the most common cause of epidural abscess in both immunocompromised and nonimmunocompromised individuals, the former are at greater risk for fungal or tuberculous abscesses. The differential diagnosis includes lymphoma, chloroma, multiple myeloma, extramedullary hematopoiesis (particularly with homogeneous enhancement), and metastatic disease. Epidural abscess is usually found in the thoracic canal because of the relatively larger volume of epidural space than in the cervical and lumbar regions, where normal cord enlargement occurs. The dorsal location within the canal is probably favored because of the paucity of ventral epidural space as a result of close approximation of the dura and posterior longitudinal ligament.

Notes

CASE 14

CSF Pulsation Artifacts

1. The patient has focal signal loss on the fast-spin-echo (FSE) T2-weighted image (left) from pulsatile CSF motion. This pseudolesion is not manifested on the low–flip angle, flow-compensated, gradient-recalled-echo (GRE) T2*-weighted image (right).

2. Gadolinium-enhanced MR angiography of the spine displays intradural vessels as hyperintense structures within the subarachnoid space.

3. Arachnoid septations in the dorsal thoracic subarachnoid space.

4. Spin saturation effect. CSF signal intensity is low on high–flip angle images because of incomplete recovery of longitudinal magnetization of the water (CSF) protons between excitations.

Reference

Pattany PM, Phillips JJ, Chiu LC, et al: Motion artifact suppression technique (MAST) for MR imaging. *J Comput Assist Tomogr* 11:369–377, 1987.

Cross-Reference

Neuroradiology: THE REQUISITES, pp 8–9.

Comment

When compared with T2*-weighted GRE images, T2-weighted FSE images are less sensitive to susceptibility effects and do not exaggerate bone-CSF or bone–soft tissue interfaces. Thus, FSE sequences are often preferred in the evaluation of patients with suspected degenerative disease of the spine. In the cervical and thoracic spine, however, relatively rapid, pulsatile CSF flow produces signal loss within the subarachnoid space, particularly on axial images, which limits the utility of FSE acquisitions. The CSF signal loss shown in the left-hand image has two potential causes. First, for FSE pulse sequences lacking flow compensation, the signal loss results from flow-induced dephasing of spins. Second, for FSE pulse sequences with flow compensation, spins that resided within the selected slice during the 90° pulse may have moved to adjacent regions by the time of the 180° pulse or may have been replaced by spins that were never exposed to the 90° pulse. For both groups of spins, no signal is generated from CSF in the selected section. This problem of motion into and out of the selected slice by flowing spins is worse for T2-weighted FSE images than for T2*-weighted GRE images because the former have much longer echo time (TE) values. In this case the GRE image was acquired with flow compensation and a TE of 18 msec, versus an effective TE of 119 msec for the FSE image.

CSF flow–induced signal loss is often less pronounced on sagittal FSE images. Signal loss is also less on axial FSE images of the lumbosacral spine than on those of the cervical spine and thoracic spine. Thus, the FSE technique is often used to acquire T2-weighted sagittal images and lumbosacral T2-weighted axial images. In the dorsal thoracic subarachnoid space, arachnoid septations that trap CSF may limit the size of areas of flow-related signal loss and produce a variable pattern of signal intensity. Septations are common in children and young adults but involute with increasing age.

Notes

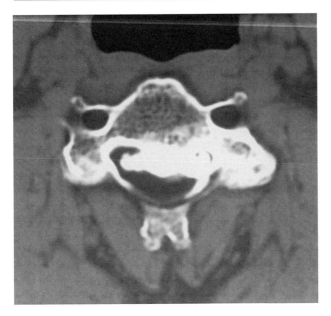

1. Is this lesion more likely to involve one vertebral level or several levels?

2. What surgical treatment, other than laminectomy, has been found efficacious?

3. Which vertebral level or levels are most severely involved?

4. What other spinal locations may show calcification in association with this lesion?

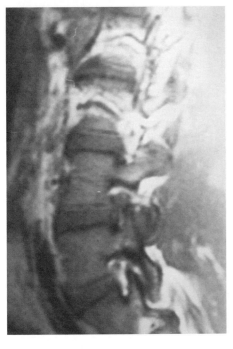

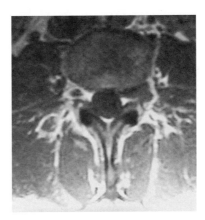

1. Based on the left parasagittal and axial (L4-5 intervertebral disk space) T1-weighted images, radiculopathy is most likely to involve which nerve root?

2. Name three types of anular tears.

3. Through which type of tear does prolapse of disk tissue most often occur?

4. Would you describe the abnormality shown here as a disk bulge, herniation, protrusion, and/or extrusion?

Ossification of the Posterior Longitudinal Ligament

1. Several levels.

2. Expansive ("open-door") laminaplasty, or laminoplasty, has been found effective in treating patients with ossification of the posterior longitudinal ligament (OPLL) and cervical myelopathy.

3. C4 through C6.

4. Ligamentum flavum and, in patients with diffuse idiopathic skeletal hyperostosis (DISH), the anterior longitudinal ligament.

Reference

Lee TT, Green BA, Gromelski EB: Safety and stability of open-door cervical expansive laminaplasty. *J Spinal Disord* 11:12-15, 1998.

Cross-Reference

Neuroradiology: THE REQUISITES, p 467.

Comment

OPLL typically involves multiple cervical levels in the midline and can show characteristic lateral extension, as illustrated in the figure. CT and plain films are probably preferable to MR imaging in identifying subtle calcification/ossification, yet MR imaging is valuable for identifying cord compression. The ossified ligament may have fatty marrow and thus increased signal on T1-weighted images. OPLL is often associated with ligamentum flavum calcification, and an association with DISH has been reported. An important finding on CT or MR images is that the calcification/ossification occurs along the length of the ligament and can thus be seen at the level of the pedicles, as shown here. This finding helps differentiate OPLL from osteophytes and calcified herniated disks, which should be present at the level of the disk space only. For patients with myelopathy, surgical treatment is aimed at decompression of the cord. In the canal-expansive laminaplasty procedure, the surgeon produces enlargement of the canal by partially resecting the lateral aspect of one lamina and then creating a hinge at the lateral aspect of the opposite lamina. The residual posterior arch is rotated about the hinge, thus opening up the canal. This procedure is usually done at each level from C3 through C7, and then bone grafts are placed across the opening at alternate levels (usually C3, C5, and C7) to keep the "door" open and the cord uncompressed.

Notes

Disk Herniation (Lateral), Lumbar

1. L4, as a result of compression in the left L4 neural foramen.

2. Concentric, transverse, and radial tears.

3. Radial tear.

4. Lateral disk herniation is a correct description. This abnormality is more likely to be an extrusion than a protrusion.

Reference

Modic MT: Degenerative disorders of the spine. In: Modic MT, Masaryk TJ, Ross JS, Eds: *Magnetic Resonance Imaging of the Spine,* second edition. St. Louis, Mosby, 1994, pp 80-150.

Cross-Reference

Neuroradiology: THE REQUISITES, pp 461-463.

Comment

Both the sagittal and axial T1-weighted images demonstrate obliteration of the normal epidural fat signal in the left neural foramen. The dorsal nerve root ganglion abuts the soft tissue mass that is contiguous with the disk. These findings indicate a left lateral (or foraminal) disk herniation with impingement on the exiting L4 nerve root. On MR and CT axial images, the disk (or anular) bulge is smooth, symmetric, and without focal protrusion. The anulus is presumed to be intact, but such may not be the case with large bulges. Disk herniations are focal and involve prolapse of the nucleus pulposus into an anular (radial) tear so that the disk extends beyond its normal anatomic margin. Disk herniations have been characterized as protrusions, extrusions, or sequestrations. In a protrusion, the anulus is presumed to be intact. This category overlaps with bulge, and differentiation depends on evidence of focality. In an extrusion, the anulus is ruptured but the posterior longitudinal ligament is intact. On cross-sectional images, extrusion is identifiable when the protruding portion ("cap") of the herniated disk is wider than the "neck" connecting the cap to the bulk of the disk in the interspace. In a sequestration, the anulus is ruptured, without or with (rare) rupture of the posterior longitudinal ligament, and a fragment of the disk becomes separated (sequestered) from the remainder of the parent disk.

Transverse and concentric tears in the anulus fibrosus of normal adult disks are common incidental findings. Radial tears develop in the inner and middle portions of the anulus fibrosus. Nuclear material prolapsing into a tear may be contained by the outer layers of the anulus or breach these layers and become extruded.

Notes

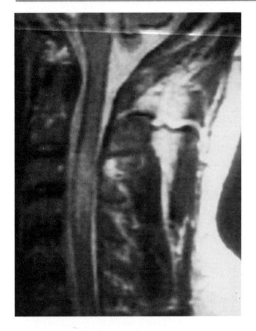
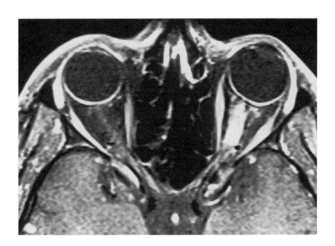

1. What syndrome is this patient likely to have?
2. Is acute orbital involvement more often unilateral or bilateral?
3. Are cerebral white matter lesions common in this syndrome?
4. With respect to cord findings, how does this syndrome differ clinically and radiologically from typical multiple sclerosis?

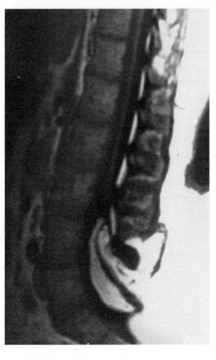
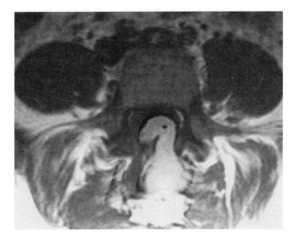

1. Which of the following terms best describe the abnormality shown on the T1-weighted axial and sagittal images of this 45-year-old woman: intradural lipoma, lipomyelomeningocele, lipomyeloschisis?
2. What is a neural placode?
3. In addition to the presence of a lipoma, how does a lipomyelomeningocele differ from a myelomeningocele?
4. Name three lesions that may preclude lumbar or cervical puncture in patients with lipomyeloschisis.

Devic's Syndrome (Neuromyelitis Optica)

1. Devic's syndrome.

2. Unilateral optic neuritis.

3. No.

4. Clinically, findings such as gait disturbance, incontinence of urine and stool, extremity weakness, sensory loss, and/or paresthesias are profound and persist after resolution of the acute disease. Radiologically, the cord is more likely to show extensive swelling and evidence of necrosis acutely and severe atrophy chronically. The findings are often more severe than the swelling and two-segment hyperintensity of the cord shown on this T2-weighted image. Postcontrast T1-weighted images of the cord should be obtained to determine whether breakdown of the blood-cord barrier has occurred, which is suggestive of necrosis.

Reference

Mandler RN, Davis LE, Jeffery DR, Kornfeld M: Devic's neuromyelitis optica: A clinicopathological study of 8 patients. *Ann Neurol* 34:162–168, 1993.

Cross-Reference

Neuroradiology: THE REQUISITES, p 206.

Comment

Devic's syndrome is characterized by rapid onset of myelopathy and optic neuropathy in the absence of CNS disease elsewhere. Myelopathy and optic neuropathy, with clinical features characteristic of transverse myelitis and optic neuritis, respectively, may occur simultaneously or be separated by weeks to months. Some authors consider Devic's syndrome a fulminant form of multiple sclerosis that progresses to severe disability or death before the appearance of plaques in other CNS regions such as cerebellar or cerebral white matter or the brainstem. Pathologically, spinal cord (gray and white matter) necrosis and cavitation and optic nerve demyelination, with or without cavitation, are present. An association of transverse myelitis and optic neuritis has been reported in other disorders such as lupus erythematosus and acute disseminated encephalomyelitis.

Notes

Lipomyelomeningocele

1. Lipomyelomeningocele and lipomyeloschisis.

2. A flat remnant of the dorsally open embryonic neural plate. The lipoma is located dorsal to the neural placode with a variable amount of intervening fibrous tissue.

3. A lipomyelomeningocele has an intact skin covering.

4. Lumbar puncture may be precluded by the presence of a low-lying conus, large lipoma, or complex lipomyelomeningocele. Cervical (C1-2) or cisternal puncture would be precluded by the presence of a Chiari II malformation with tonsillar ectopia.

Reference

Sutton LN: Lipomyelomeningocele. *Neurosurg Clin N Am* 6:325–338, 1995.

Cross-Reference

Neuroradiology: THE REQUISITES, pp 273–274.

Comment

Lipomyelomeningocele is distinguished from intradural lipoma by the presence of a widely bifid spinal canal and protrusion of lipoma and dural sac through the defect. Lipomyeloschisis is a term that encompasses both lesions and refers to a spectrum of conditions characterized by variable protrusion of a lipoma into the associated dorsal dysraphic defect. Lipomyelomeningoceles have been classified, for the purpose of surgical management, into those that insert caudally into the conus and those that attach to the dorsal surface of the conus. In the former, which is exemplified by this case, the lipoma may replace the filum terminale, or a separate filum may lie anteriorly. The nerve roots usually lie ventral to the lipoma. In this case, lobulation of the lipoma and rotation of the neural placode have resulted in a complex-appearing lesion with cord tethering and a low position of the conus.

Notes

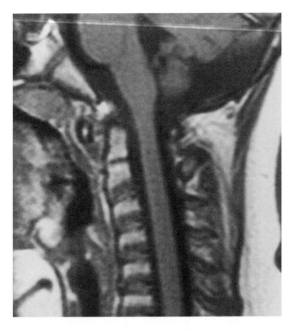 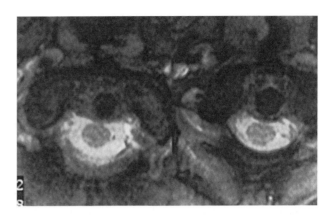

1. Is the atlantoaxial articulation normal in this 8-year-old boy (sagittal T1-weighted and axial T2*-weighted images)?

2. What is the primary motion at C1-2?

3. In children with craniovertebral injury, is odontoid fracture or transverse ligament rupture more likely to occur?

4. How does the distribution of posttraumatic cervical spinal cord injury in adults compare with the distribution in children?

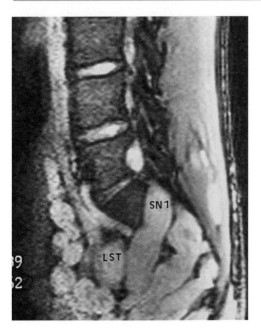

1. Name three conditions that may cause diffuse peripheral nerve enlargement.

2. What nerves primarily contribute to the lumbosacral trunk?

3. What is the typical composition of the sacral plexus?

4. What are the two classic types of neurofibroma?

Atlantoaxial Subluxation

1. The atlantodental distance appears abnormally large, and effacement of the ventral subarachnoid space is present; however, proper evaluation under current guidelines should include flexion-extension lateral radiographs and CT scans to screen for fractures and assess stability.

2. Rotation.

3. In children, rupture of the transverse ligament is rare.

4. Adults tend to have lower cervical cord injuries, whereas children tend to have upper cervical cord injuries.

References

Bonadio WA: Cervical spine trauma in children, Part I. General concepts, normal anatomy, radiographic evaluation. *Am J Emerg Med* 11:158–165, 1993.

Bonadio WA: Cervical spine trauma in children, Part II. Mechanisms and manifestations of injury, therapeutic considerations. *Am J Emerg Med* 11:256–278, 1993.

Cross-Reference

Neuroradiology: THE REQUISITES, p 501.

Comment

Much has been written about the pitfalls in interpretation of atlantoaxial subluxation and instability in children. The transverse ligament crosses behind the odontoid process and inserts on the inner margin of the C1 ring laterally, thus restricting the anterior-posterior motion of C1 relative to C2.

In children, especially those younger than 8 years, ligamentous laxity results in a larger range of motion. Thus, the maximum atlantodental distance (distance between the posterior margin of the anterior arch of C1 and the dens) is usually taken to be 5 mm, versus 3 mm in adults. Ostensibly, greater laxity reduces the frequency of transverse ligament rupture and therefore places the odontoid at greater risk of fracture when a force is applied to the craniovertebral/upper cervical region.

This boy, who was hit by a car while skateboarding, had CT and plain radiography, including flexion and extension views. The atlantodental distance was 5 mm by CT and ranged from 3 mm in extension to 8 mm in flexion on lateral radiographs. No fractures were seen. In addition to the MR imaging findings just described, moderate narrowing of the dorsal subarachnoid space was noted, but no cord compression. No abnormal signal was detected in the spinal cord or in the region of the transverse ligament. Based on the clinical and imaging results, the neurosurgeon performed a C1-C2 posterior fusion with cerclage wires and bone graft.

Notes

Sacral Neurofibromas (Neurofibromatosis Type 1)

1. Neurofibromatosis type 1 (NF1), Dejerine-Sottas disease, and Charcot-Marie-Tooth disease.

2. L4 and L5.

3. Anterior rami of L4 through S4.

4. Plexiform and dermal.

Reference

Wiestler OD, Radner H: Pathology of neurofibromatosis 1 and 2. In: Huson SM, Hughes RAC, Eds: *The Neurofibromatoses: A Pathogenetic and Clinical Overview.* New York, Chapman & Hall, 1994, pp 135–159.

Cross-Reference

Neuroradiology: THE REQUISITES, p 490.

Comment

Neurofibromas are spindle cell neoplasms that arise from a peripheral nerve sheath. They contain a mixture of Schwann cells and perineurial fibroblasts and are the hallmark of NF1, an autosomal dominant disorder mapped to chromosome 17. Classically, two variants of neurofibroma are observed in NF1, dermal neurofibroma and plexiform neurofibroma. Dermal neurofibromas originate from terminal nerve branches in the skin and are not associated with major peripheral nerve trunks. Plexiform neurofibromas, which originate from subcutaneous and visceral peripheral nerves and nerve roots, often exhibit marked intrafascicular growth. Tumor cells intermixed with collagen are embedded in an abundant extracellular myxoid matrix. The fascicular organization of the affected nerve is maintained, yet individual fascicles may become enlarged by the intrafascicular neoplasm to such an extent that together they resemble a nerve plexus (hence "plexiform" neurofibroma). Enlargement of the nerve produces a fusiform appearance or irregular cylindric shape. Typically, multiple nerves are involved, as shown in this case of sacral nerve root and plexus involvement.

When compared with schwannomas (neurilemomas), which are composed of only Schwann cells, neurofibromas usually exhibit significant amounts of extracellular collagen, as well as myelinated and unmyelinated axons. In addition, neurofibromas have a relative lack of hemorrhage and degenerative change. Although typically solitary, schwannomas may occur at multiple sites in individuals with NF2 (mapped to chromosome 22).

On MR imaging, neurofibromas and schwannomas can be indistinguishable and are thus considered under the heading of nerve sheath tumors in the differential diagnosis of a mass or enlargement involving a peripheral nerve. Diffuse, elongated, or fusiform enlargement of multiple nerves, as in this case (LST, lumbosacral trunk; SN1, ventral ramus of the first sacral nerve; SN2 and SN3 are unlabeled), favors neurofibromas in an individual with NF1. These tumors often show central areas of hypointensity on T2-weighted images, presumably because of dense collagen intermixed with proliferations of tumor cells. Peripheral hyperintensity is attributed to the surrounding myxoid matrix. Larger tumors (>5 cm) have more variable signal intensity centrally as a result of necrosis.

Notes

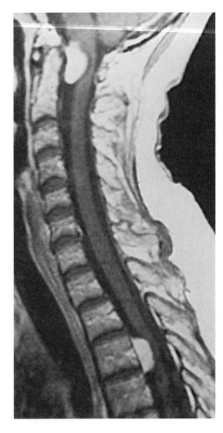

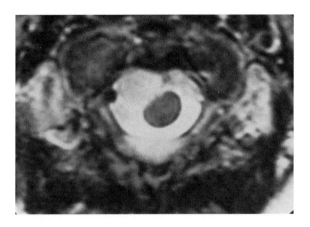

1. What is the most common tumor of the foramen magnum?

2. A T2-weighted fast-spin-echo axial image (C1-2 level) and a postcontrast T1-weighted sagittal image of the cervical spine are shown in this case. What imaging study could be diagnostic?

3. How does lesion location along the spinal axis influence your differential diagnosis?

4. Name two intramedullary lesions that should be looked for in this case.

Multiple Meningiomas, Cervicothoracic

1. Meningioma.

2. Postcontrast T1-weighted images of the internal auditory canals that demonstrate bilateral acoustic schwannomas are diagnostic of neurofibromatosis type 2 (NF2).

3. The favored sites for spinal meningioma are the cervicomedullary junction and thoracic region, as in this case.

4. Syringomyelia and ependymoma.

Reference

Mautner VF, Tatagiba M, Lindenau M, et al: Spinal tumors in patients with neurofibromatosis type 2: MR imaging study of frequency, multiplicity, and variety. *AJR Am J Roentgenol* 165:951–955, 1995.

Cross-Reference

Neuroradiology: THE REQUISITES, pp 267–268, 489–490.

Comment

The postcontrast T1-weighted sagittal image demonstrates two similar, extramedullary-intradural lesions, each having a broad base on the dura and causing cord compression. The differential diagnosis includes meningioma, nerve sheath tumor, and metastasis. Meningioma is favored because of location at the foramen magnum and in the thoracic spine, where 80% of meningiomas are found. The mass is located anterior-lateral to the cord and is hyperintense relative to the cord on the axial T2-weighted image. The hyperintensity favors schwannoma over meningioma; however, several authors have noticed that increased signal is not uncommon in meningiomas. In reporting the findings on the axial image, it is important to comment on the location of the vertebral arteries relative to the mass for the benefit of the surgeon. Both meningiomas and nerve sheath tumors of the size shown here exhibit striking enhancement and sharp margins on postcontrast images. Compression of the cord, especially at the foramen magnum, should prompt a search for syringomyelia.

The occurrence of multiple meningiomas is rare and is associated with NF2. Patients with NF2 are also at risk for intramedullary (ependymoma) and other extramedullary (schwannoma, neurofibroma) lesions. In one study, 82% of patients (n = 73) with NF2 had intradural-extramedullary tumors on MR imaging. These tumors could not be differentiated on the basis of signal intensity or postcontrast enhancement. Based on histologic findings in about one fourth of the patients, the tumors were schwannomas, meningiomas, and neurofibromas (in order of frequency). The schwannomas were usually found in the lumbar region.

Notes

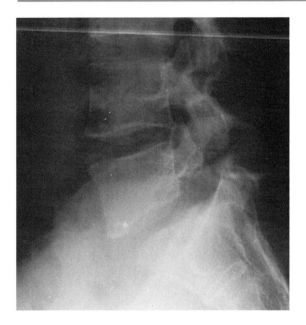

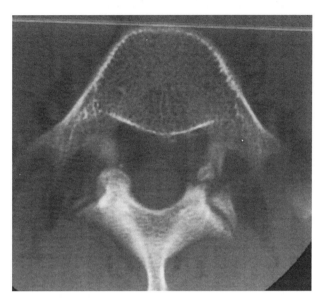

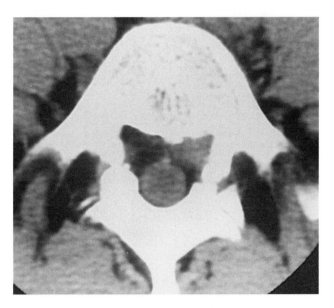

1. Differentiate spondylolisthesis from spondylolysis.

2. Is the frequency of spina bifida increased in the population with spondylolisthesis?

3. Is disk herniation more common at the level of the spondylolisthesis or immediately above it?

4. Does this 25-year-old man with low back pain and no history of trauma have a "pseudoherniation" on the axial CT images?

Isthmic (Spondylolytic) Spondylolisthesis

1. Spondylolisthesis refers to anterior slippage of a vertebra relative to the subjacent vertebra, whereas spondylolysis refers to a defect, congenital or acquired, in the pars interarticularis, which may or may not be associated with vertebral slippage.

2. Spina bifida of L5, as well as spina bifida of S1, is associated with two types of spondylolisthesis—congenital (dysplastic) and isthmic.

3. The level immediately above the spondylolisthesis.

4. No, it is real because it is focal and has a left paracentral (or subarticular) location.

References

Amundson G, Edwards CC, Garfin SR: Spondylolisthesis. In: Herkowitz HN, Garfin SR, Balderston RA, et al, Eds: *The Spine,* fourth edition. Philadelphia, WB Saunders, 1999, pp 835–885.

Rothman SLG, Glenn WV Jr: CT multiplanar reconstruction in 253 cases of lumbar spondylolysis. *AJNR Am J Neuroradiol* 5:81–90, 1984.

Cross-Reference

Neuroradiology: THE REQUISITES, pp 459, 468.

Comment

The lateral radiograph demonstrates anterior slippage, or subluxation, of L5 on S1. The slippage is one fourth or less of the vertebral body width and is therefore termed grade 1 spondylolisthesis. On the bone window image at the L5-S1 level can be seen bilateral defects in the bony canal. These defects involve the isthmus (pars interarticularis) on each side of the L5 vertebra. Thus, bilateral spondylolysis of L5 is present. Note that the pars defects have a more horizontal orientation than do the L5-S1 facet joints, which are obliquely orientated and located more posteriorly. The anterior slippage of L5 on S1 is referred to as isthmic (spondylolytic) spondylolisthesis in the widely accepted classification of Newman. This classification differentiates five types of spondylolistheses, and a sixth type has been added since Newman's description was published: (I) congenital (dysplastic), (II) isthmic (spondylolytic), (III) degenerative, (IV) traumatic, (V) pathologic, and (VI) postsurgical. For type II, the isthmic defect probably results from a combination of hereditary dysplasia of the pars interarticularis, stress imposed on the lower lumbar spine by an upright bipedal posture, and extension loading (repeated microfractures leaving the pars elongated).

The axial image with a soft tissue window and level shows a left paracentral extradural mass representing an L5-S1 herniated disk. This focal mass differs in appearance from a "pseudoherniation," which on axial images is an apparent (rather than real) broad protrusion of the disk margin posterior to the margin of the slipped vertebral body. True disk herniation at the level of the spondylolisthesis is unusual.

Notes

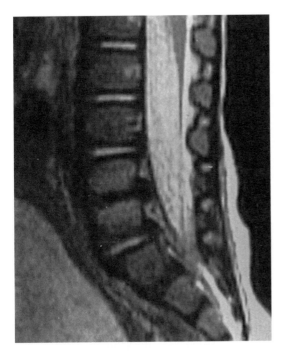
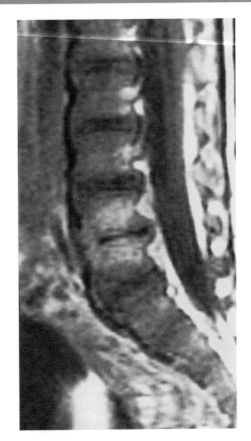

1. For the disorder shown on the fast-spin-echo T2-weighted image and the postcontrast T1-weighted image, list the expected sites of involvement (cervical, thoracic, lumbar) in children in descending order.

2. What finding is atypical for this disorder?

3. Where did the pathologic changes in the spine probably begin in this 1½-year-old girl?

4. Is involvement of the pedicle, transverse process, and/or spinous process more likely in pyogenic or tuberculous spondylitis?

Diskitis/Osteomyelitis, Pediatric

1. Lumbar > thoracic > cervical.

2. Low signal intensity within the disk space at L4-5 on the T2-weighted image.

3. In a child, infection begins either in the disk space or in the anterior subchondral space (end-plate), whereas in an adult, infection begins in the subchondral space.

4. Tuberculosis.

Reference

Song KS, Ogden JA, Ganey T, Guidera KJ: Contiguous discitis and osteomyelitis in children. *J Pediatr Orthop* 17:470–477, 1997.

Cross-Reference

Neuroradiology: THE REQUISITES, pp 477–478.

Comment

This child had a urinary tract infection that was treated with antibiotics 2 weeks before admission for fever and difficulty ambulating. Findings typical of osteomyelitis/diskitis at L4-5 are increased signal intensity within the bodies of L4 and L5 on the T2-weighted image and postcontrast enhancement within the bodies and the intervertebral disk space on the postcontrast T1-weighted image. Another typical finding, enhancement of the prevertebral and epidural soft tissues at the involved level, is present at L4-5 but not well shown on the T1-weighted image without fat suppression. Low signal intensity within the involved disk space is less common than high signal intensity and may be related to previous antibiotic treatment.

In adults, spondylitis resulting from hematogenous dissemination of infection begins in the anterior subchondral space of the vertebral end-plate. This space is favored because of its rich vascularization and termination of the vascular tree in this region. Children have a residual blood supply to the disk, so diskitis may precede osteomyelitis. From a nidus in the subchondral space, infection may spread (1) into the disk space and from there to the adjacent vertebral body, (2) anteriorly into the subligamentous space and from there to adjacent vertebral bodies or to the paraspinal soft tissues, or (3) posteriorly into the same vertebra. Preferred directions of spread have been interpreted in terms of aggressiveness of the infection. Pyogenic spondylitis (more aggressive) almost always attacks the disk space, whereas tuberculous spondylitis (more indolent) has "time to spread" anteriorly to the subligamentous space or posteriorly into the vertebra with relative sparing of the disk space sometimes.

Notes

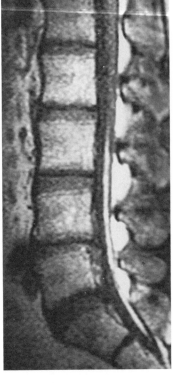
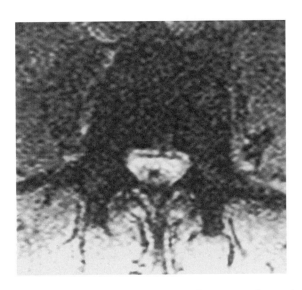

1. What is the prevalence in normal adults of the intradural lesion shown on the sagittal T1-weighted spin-echo and axial T2*-weighted gradient-echo images?
2. In what other lumbosacral location is this lesion found?
3. Define "tight filum terminale syndrome."
4. What congenital anomalies are strongly associated with this syndrome?

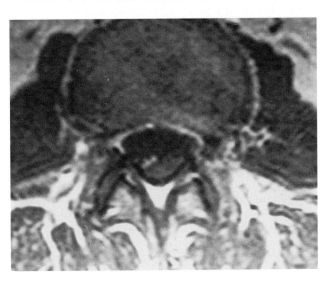
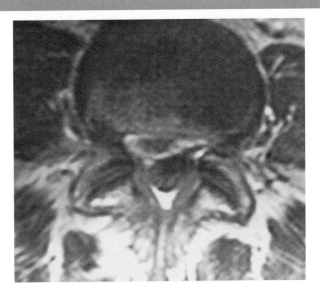

1. Postcontrast (0.1 mmol/kg gadolinium chelate) T1-weighted axial images were obtained at the levels of L3 (left image) and L4-5 (right image) in a 62-year-old woman with right lower extremity pain. How common is lumbar nerve root enhancement in unoperated patients?
2. What two degenerative conditions seem to be associated with this enhancement?
3. What normal structures may mimic an enhancing nerve root?
4. What AIDS-related opportunistic infection is often manifested as lumbosacral nerve root enhancement?

Lipoma of the Filum Terminale

1. Lipoma (or fibrolipoma) of the filum has been found incidentally in 4% to 6% of normal adults on postmortem examination.

2. Lipoma can be intradural, extradural, or both.

3. Thickened (>2 mm in diameter) filum with a tethered conus (tip below L2 in 86% of cases).

4. Midline defects in the arches of the lumbosacral spine, especially L4, L5, and/or S1.

Reference

Brown E, Matthes JC, Bazan C 3rd, Jinkins JR: Prevalence of incidental intraspinal lipoma of the lumbosacral spine as determined by MRI. *Spine* 19:833–836, 1994.

Cross-Reference

Neuroradiology: THE REQUISITES, p 275.

Comment

The images are from a 39-year-old man with recent onset of left sciatica. The filum is thickened, has high signal intensity on the T1-weighted image, and has low signal intensity on the T2*-weighted image, consistent with fat. The conus is in a normal position with its tip at L1-2 (confirmed on axial images) and without evidence of tethering. These findings may be considered a normal variation because of their incidental occurrence in normal adults. Multiple congenital anomalies, however, occur in association with a thickened filum (with or without fat), especially when the conus is tethered. The subcutaneous fat, lumbar fascia, and posterior spinal elements, in particular, must be carefully evaluated for evidence of dysraphic lesions.

Some authors refer to a more focal, fusiform enlargement of the filum as a filar lipoma and distinguish it from the diffusely thickened fatty filum shown here. Note that the patient has a herniated disk at L4-5. This disk protruded into the left anterior epidural space and was considered to be responsible for the recent sciatica.

Notes

Enhancing Nerve Roots With Lumbar Disk Herniation (Unoperated Spine)

1. Probably about 5%, presuming that enhancing medullary veins are distinguished from enhancing roots.

2. Spinal stenosis and disk herniation.

3. Intradural medullary veins and the sacral dorsal root ganglia.

4. Cytomegalovirus polyradiculitis.

References

Jinkins JR: MR of nerve root enhancement in the unoperated lumbosacral spine. *AJNR Am J Neuroradiol* 14:193–202, 1993.

Lane JI, Koeller KK, Atkinson LD: Enhanced lumbar nerve roots in the spine without prior surgery: Radiculitis or radicular veins? *AJNR Am J Neuroradiol* 15:1317–1325, 1994.

Cross-Reference

Neuroradiology: THE REQUISITES, pp 472–474.

Comment

In this patient with no history of previous spine surgery, the image at the level of L3 shows punctate enhancement along the right side of the cauda equina. At the level of L4-5 can be seen punctate enhancement posterior to the enhancing rim of a right paracentral herniated disk. By tracking the punctate enhancement on contiguous axial images and on sagittal images, the punctate enhancing structures were tentatively identified as the right L4 and L5 nerve roots.

The prevalence of abnormal enhancement of lumbosacral nerve roots in unoperated patients with low back pain and/or radiculopathy is reported to be about 5%, with associated focal disk protrusion in the majority (70%) of these cases. The results have been disputed, though, by one group of investigators, who reported a higher prevalence (25%) but attributed it to enhancing medullary (sometimes called radiculomedullary or radicular) veins and found a poor correlation between enhancement and clinical radiculopathy. In theory, the large medullary veins, which drain from the midline anterior or posterior median veins on the conus, should be distinguishable from enhancing nerve roots, which originate more laterally from the cord surface. For sacral nerves, the sensory ganglia, which lack a blood-nerve barrier (BNB), are located within the sacral canal along the course of the dorsal root. Thus, normal enhancement of these ganglia may mimic pathologic enhancement in the sacral region. Pathologic enhancement of the remainder of the sacral nerve roots and the lumbar roots in the cauda equina has been attributed to a breakdown of the BNB of these roots resulting from a variety of nonspecific insults—compression, ischemia, inflammation, active demyelination, or axonal degeneration.

Notes

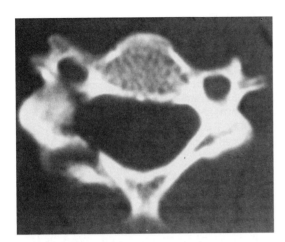
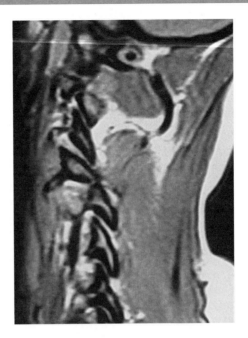

1. Which findings on the axial CT image (C4 level) characterize this type of fracture?
2. Which finding on the right parasagittal T1-weighted MR image is consistent with this type of fracture?
3. What is the probable mechanism of injury?
4. Can this fracture be stabilized by one-level plating?

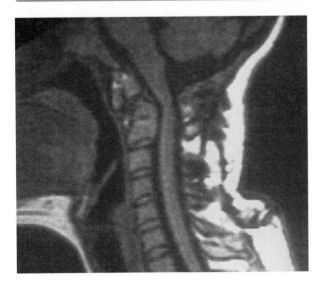
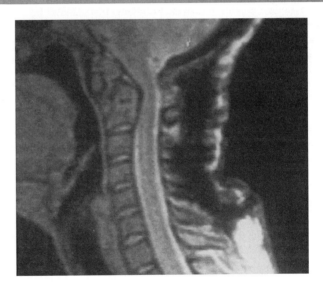

1. How does ossiculum terminale differ from os odontoideum?
2. Can the diagnosis of ossiculum terminale be made in children?
3. What features may help distinguish congenital os odontoideum from an old odontoid fracture with nonunion?
4. What does the horizontal dark line seen within C2 on the T1- and T2*-weighted sagittal images represent?

C A S E 2 6

Fracture-Separation of the Articular Mass

1. Fractures through the right lamina and the right pedicle.

2. "Horizontalization" of the right lateral mass.

3. Extension-rotation.

4. No.

Reference

Levine AM: Facet fractures and dislocations. In: Levine AM, Eismont FJ, Garfin SR, Zigler JE, Eds: *Spine Trauma*. Philadelphia, WB Saunders, 1998, pp 331–366.

Cross-Reference

Neuroradiology: THE REQUISITES, p 500.

Comment

As evidenced by the rotation of the C4 vertebra on the CT image and by the offset of the facets on the parasagittal MR image, this is a unilateral facet injury. These injuries are categorized as purely ligamentous (ranging from facet subluxation to "perched facet" to facet dislocation), as distinct fractures of the superior facet or inferior facet, or as fracture-separations of the articular mass with associated displacement. The fractures through the right lamina and the pedicle identify this injury as a fracture-separation of the right lateral mass. This fracture is more often seen as a unilateral injury than a bilateral injury. The mechanism is extension-rotation, as opposed to the flexion-rotation responsible for superior or inferior facet fractures. The fracture-separation creates a free-floating fragment with rotational instability that cannot be stabilized over a single level but rather requires stabilization at both C4-5 and C3-4. Typically, treatment is bilateral lateral mass plating from C3 through C5 (two level, C3-4 and C4-5). After fracturing, the lateral mass often rotates, and lateral radiographs, or a parasagittal MR image (as here), may show "horizontalization" of the lateral mass. Correspondingly, the anterior-posterior radiograph shows foreshortening of the lateral mass. In this case, horizontalization and displacement of the right C4 lateral mass have resulted in perching of the tip of the inferior articular process (here referred to as the inferior facet) of C4 on the superior articular process of C5.

Notes

C A S E 2 7

Os Odontoideum

1. Ossiculum terminale results from failure of the apical portion of the dens to fuse with the body of the dens, whereas os odontoideum results from failure of the combined apical plus basal portions of the dens to fuse with the body of C2.

2. The diagnosis can be made in children older than 12 years, by which time the normal apical ossification center of the odontoid will have fused with the base of the dens.

3. Congenital and "acquired" (posttraumatic) os odontoideum may be indistinguishable; however, in the congenital anomaly the os is often smaller than the normal odontoid, has a rounded contour, and is separated from the odontoid base by a wide gap rather than a thin fracture line.

4. This line is the synchondrosis at the odontoid base.

Reference

Smoker WR: Craniovertebral junction: Normal anatomy, craniometry, and congenital anomalies. *Radiographics* 14:255–277, 1994.

Cross-Reference

Neuroradiology: THE REQUISITES, pp 450, 501.

Comment

The normal odontoid process develops from three ossification centers, two primary and one secondary. If these centers unite but fail to fuse with the body of C2, the result is a congenital os odontoideum, which is located posterior and superior to the anterior arch of C1. Anterior displacement of the os-atlas complex relative to the body of the axis in the neutral lateral position, as well as increased range of motion (instability) during flexion and extension, may result in cord compression, as shown in this case. The sharp irregular lines of an acute type II dens fracture are easily distinguished from the smooth, sclerotic margins of os odontoideum; however, it may be impossible to differentiate congenital os odontoideum from an old fracture.

Notes

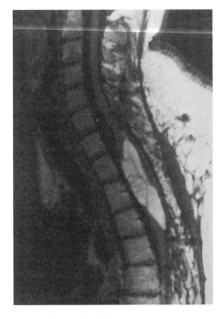
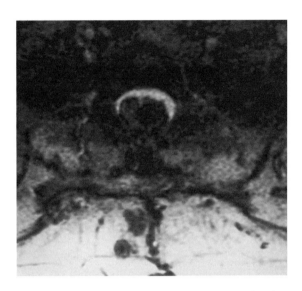

1. In this patient with previous laminectomy the T1-weighted sagittal and T2*-weighted axial images show an intramedullary mass with signal characteristics of what type of tissue?

2. Why is the left side of the cord darker on the axial gradient-echo image?

3. The tumor shown here is most frequently found in which spinal region: cervical, thoracic, or lumbar?

4. Where would you expect to find the dorsal nerve roots relative to the mass?

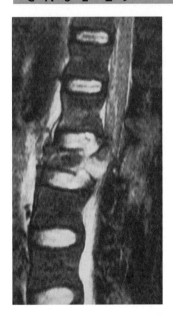
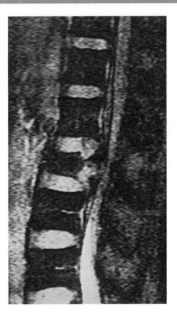

1. Is this a compression fracture or a burst fracture of L2? What is the primary difference between these two types of injury?

2. The T2-weighted fast-spin-echo (FSE) and T2*-weighted gradient-recalled-echo (GRE) images shown here were obtained within 12 hours of injury. What pathologic processes primarily account for the MR signal changes within an acutely compressed vertebral body?

3. What would you tell the referring clinician regarding cord compression in this case?

4. How would you account for the differences in these two images?

Intradural Lipoma, Thoracic

1. Adipose tissue.

2. The darker color may be due to the shorter T2 relaxation time of fat versus cord and/or an "out-of-phase" cancellation effect of the water and lipid signals in voxels containing cord adjacent to or infiltrated by lipoma.

3. The most frequent location for intradural lipomas is the thoracic region (about 30% of cases).

4. Lateral to the ventral roots and anterior to the cord-lipoma junction.

References

DeLaPaz RL: Congenital anomalies of the spine and spinal cord. In: Enzmann DR, DeLaPaz RL, Rubin JB, Eds: *Magnetic Resonance of the Spine*. St. Louis, Mosby, 1990, pp 176–236.

Razack N, Jimenez OF, Aldana P, Ragheb J: Intramedullary holocord lipoma in an athlete: Case report. *Neurosurgery* 42:394–396, 1998.

Cross-Reference

Neuroradiology: THE REQUISITES, p 490.

Comment

The intradural and apparently intramedullary mass extending from T1 to T3 is hyperintense on the T1-weighted image and hypointense on the T2*-weighted image relative to cord tissue, consistent with a lipoma. Lobules, which result from subdivision of the tumor by connective tissue strands, are evident. While the term "intradural" is routinely used, it has been noted that these tumors usually have some connection with the dorsal thecal sac and are thus not completely intradural. They may appear to be intramedullary, as in this case. In accordance with the hypothesis of premature dysjunction, however, a boundary separates the dorsally placed lipoma from the cord proper, and this arrangement results in splaying of the dorsal horns (myeloschisis) and an anterior-lateral course of the dorsal roots (analogous to the findings reported for lipomyelomeningocele). Hypothetically, the dorsal roots should be distinct from the tumor; however, dorsal roots exiting through the lateral aspect of the lipoma have been observed, and this condition plus the lack of a distinct plane between the tumor and the spinal cord may preclude complete resection of the tumor. Cases such as this one, in which the lipoma appears to encompass the entire cross section of the cord at some level, represent about 3% of all cases of intradural lipoma. Despite the appearance, an attenuated neural placode bordered by the larger lipoma is present, and the tumor does not actually replace cord. Intradural lipomas account for approximately 1% of primary intraspinal masses. Most (55%) are discovered in individuals between 10 and 30 years of age. Enlargement of the spinal canal (with associated erosion of pedicles, lamina, and/or vertebral body) is the most commonly associated vertebral abnormality and is detected in 53% of cases.

Notes

Burst Fracture With Acute Epidural Hematoma, Lumbar

1. Disruption of the posterior wall or margin of the vertebral body, as in this case, occurs with a burst fracture and not with a compression fracture.

2. Interstitial edema and hemorrhage.

3. The patient has compression of the conus at T12 and L1 by an epidural hematoma and compression at the conus–cauda equina junction by the retropulsed bone from L2.

4. Greater sensitivity of the gradient-echo images to susceptibility effects resulting from acute hemorrhage (deoxyhemoglobin) and bone fragments in the canal.

References

Levine AM: Classification of spinal injury. In: Levine AM, Eismont FJ, Garfin SR, Zigler JE, Eds: *Spine Trauma*. Philadelphia, WB Saunders, 1998, pp 113–132.

Sklar EM, Post JM, Falcone S: MRI of acute spinal epidural hematomas. *J Comput Assist Tomogr* 23:238–243, 1999.

Cross-Reference

Neuroradiology: THE REQUISITES, p 501.

Comment

Both images demonstrate decreased height of the L2 body with mixed signal intensity of the retropulsed bone from the burst fracture. The Denis classification of burst fractures is often used to describe these injuries and relate them to the mechanism of the injury and the appropriate orthopedic treatment. Increased signal within the retropulsed bone is most likely due to increased free water in the bone marrow from edema and possibly hemorrhage. No disk herniation is seen in this case.

At T12 and L1, above the level of the fracture, loss of the normal CSF hyperintensity surrounding the conus medullaris can be noted. An area that is isointense relative to cord on the T2-weighted FSE image is anterior to the conus. The GRE image is particularly helpful in delineating the area, which has features of an acute epidural hematoma and extends from T12 through L3. The increased sensitivity of GRE images, both axial and sagittal, in detecting acute epidural and subdural spinal hematomas has been reported by several investigators and attributed to the presence of low–signal intensity paramagnetic deoxyhemoglobin in these collections (abutting low–signal intensity dura). With spin-echo MR imaging, acute spinal epidural hematomas are typically isointense to hyperintense relative to cord on T1-weighted images and hyperintense with areas of hypointensity on T2-weighted images. Capping of epidural fat, direct continuity with adjacent osseous structures, and compression of epidural fat, the subarachnoid sac, and the spinal cord are common findings. Acute spinal epidural hematomas occurring in the absence of trauma or after minor (or unrelated) trauma have been observed in patients with coagulopathy, spinal arteriovenous malformation, vertebral body hemangioma, hypertension, or pregnancy. The procedures most often implicated in the formation of acute epidural hematoma are lumbar puncture and spinal anesthesia.

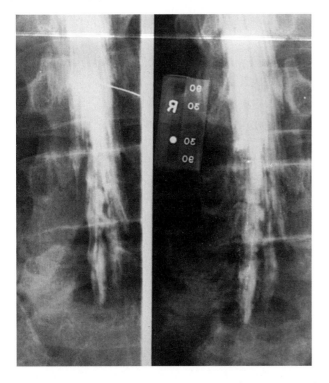

1. Name five noninfectious causes for the myelographic features in the figure.

2. A classification of the variable appearance of lumbar arachnoiditis on CT myelography and MR imaging identifies three groups or patterns. What are they?

3. Under what conditions is central clumping of nerve roots of the cauda equina reversible, based on MR imaging?

4. True or false: In the majority of cases, little enhancement of arachnoiditis is seen on post-contrast MR imaging.

Arachnoiditis

1. Carcinomatous meningitis, lymphoma, neurofibromas, Dejerine-Sottas syndrome, and spinal arteriovenous malformation.

2. Pattern 1 is clumping of nerve roots into cords and represents central adhesion of the roots within the thecal sac. Pattern 2 is referred to as the empty thecal sac sign and represents adhesion of the nerve roots to the meninges. In pattern 3, the end stage of the inflammatory response, the thecal sac is filled by a mass. On myelography this stage produces a block to the flow of intrathecal contrast material, with an irregular "candle-dripping" appearance.

3. Reversible clumping after lumbar laminectomy has been described.

4. True.

Reference

Delamarter RB, Ross JS, Masaryk TJ, Modic MT, Bohlman HH: Diagnosis of lumbar arachnoiditis by magnetic resonance imaging. *Spine* 15:304–310, 1990.

Cross-Reference

Neuroradiology: THE REQUISITES, p 473.

Comment

With the advent of MR imaging, the use of myelography with iodinated intrathecal contrast for the diagnosis of intraspinal disease has decreased dramatically. Patients with magnetically sensitive devices, such as cardiac pacemakers, and some patients with spinal instrumentation, such as rods, screws, or wires with or without ferromagnetic properties, still require myelography for diagnosis. In lumbar myelography, the normal lumbosacral roots of the cauda equina have a thin feathery pattern, with contrast material filling the thecal sac and surrounding each root. In patients with arachnoiditis or arachnoidal adhesions from a variety of causes, thickening and clumping of the roots can produce incomplete filling of the sac and an irregular, beaded appearance of the contrast column, as shown in this case. This degree of clumping would probably result in a pattern 1 appearance of the cauda equina on axial images from CT myelography or MR imaging studies. This appearance may be indistinguishable from drop metastases, although the latter are said to be less smooth, less symmetric, and more irregular and to demonstrate greater enhancement on postcontrast T1-weighted MR images. For pattern 2 arachnoiditis, standard myelography and CT myelography demonstrate homogeneous, featureless filling of the distal thecal sac, without visible nerve roots. MR images have a similar appearance, although the clumped nerve roots adherent to the meninges may be visible. Causes of arachnoiditis include infection, subarachnoid hemorrhage (secondary to trauma, surgery, or vascular malformation), and inflammatory diseases (e.g., sarcoidosis).

Notes

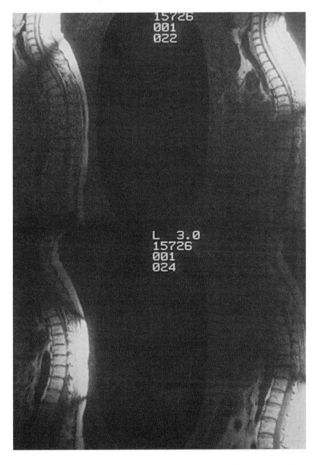

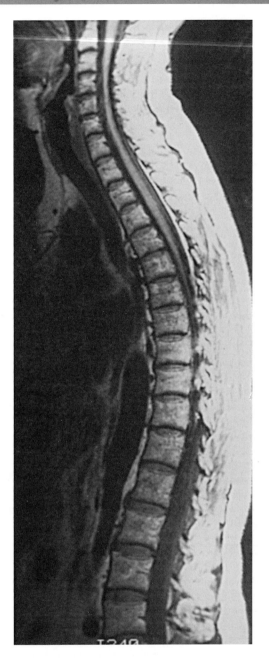

1. What type of radiofrequency coil is being used as a receiver for the MR signal—a volume coil or a surface coil?

2. Why do we use this type of coil for spinal imaging?

3. What coil configuration has been used to produce the single image (right) encompassing almost the entire spine?

4. What is the major advantage of this type of configuration?

Phased-Array Coil (Multicoil) System

1. Surface coil.

2. Because a small surface coil gives a relatively high MR signal-to-noise ratio (SNR) close to the coil. For a circular-loop surface coil, the best SNR is obtained when the diameter of the loop is approximately equal to the depth of the region of interest.

3. Phased array.

4. It collects data simultaneously from a distribution of surface coils to achieve the SNR of a surface coil with the field of view (FOV) of a volume coil.

Reference

Roemer PB, Edelstein WA, Hayes CE, Souza SP, Mueller OM: The NMR phased array. *Magn Reson Med* 16:192–225, 1990.

Cross-Reference

Neuroradiology: THE REQUISITES, pp 10–11.

Comment

The first figure shows four T1-weighted images with high SNRs successively displaying the cervical, upper thoracic, lower thoracic, and lumbar regions. These images were obtained with a linear array of four surface coils located along the back. By turning only the first (uppermost) coil on, an image of the cervical spine is produced. By turning only the second coil on, an image of the upper thoracic spine is produced, and so forth. When the coils are combined as a phased array, all are "turned on" and the images are acquired simultaneously. Each voxel in the spine region induces a signal in each coil that varies in both phase and amplitude, depending on the relative location of the voxel and the coil. After the signal amplitudes are appropriately weighted and the signal phases for the different coils are adjusted to a common value, the signals are added constructively to produce a single, relatively uniform intensity image of almost the entire spine (image on the right).

A distinction is usually made between volume coils (head or body coil), which are designed to surround the region being imaged, and surface coils, which are intended to fit closely over some specific anatomic region (spine or temporomandibular joint coil). Spine imaging with conventional rectangular surface coils used to be time-consuming because conventional coils had to be repositioned and the scan repeated at several locations along the spine. This technique is no longer necessary with the spinal phased array. Because the signals received by adjacent coils in the array can be combined constructively, phased-array coils provide a twofold or threefold increase in SNR at the usual depth of the spine. These coils also produce increased uniformity in signal with depth and with distance along the length of the spine. The typical spinal phased array allows acquisition of a 48-cm linear FOV in a single imaging period and yields a high-resolution image, as shown in the image on the right.

Notes

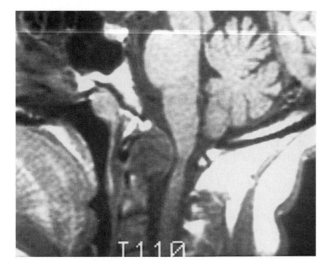

1. Name three inflammatory conditions associated with atlantoaxial dislocation.
2. How would you distinguish between joint effusion and pannus in patients with rheumatoid arthritis of the craniocervical region?
3. What are the five possible subluxations/dislocations at the C1-2 level, and which one is most common?
4. What is the importance of identifying the supradental fat pad?

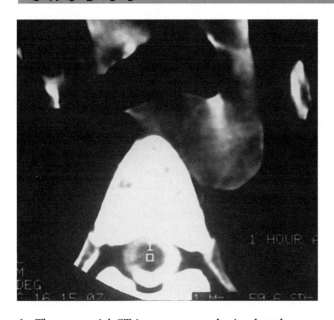
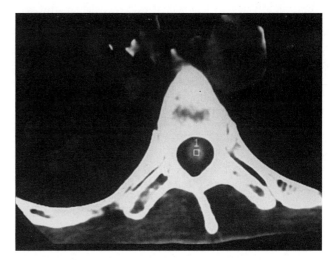

1. The two axial CT images were obtained at the same spinal level and on the same day with the same technique. Why are they different?
2. Describe a possible etiology for syringomyelia.
3. Distinguish between hydromyelia and syringomyelia.
4. Which is associated with congenital spinal and hindbrain anomalies?

Adult Rheumatoid Arthritis

1. Rheumatoid arthritis, ankylosing spondylitis, and tonsillitis/pharyngitis.

2. Contrast-enhanced T1-weighted spin-echo MR images.

3. Anterior, posterior, lateral, rotary, and vertical. Anterior is most common.

4. In patients with rheumatoid arthritis, loss of supradental fat implies the presence of pannus and/or thickened ligaments.

References

Bundschuh C, Modic MT, Kearney F, Morris R, Deal C: Rheumatoid arthritis of the cervical spine: Surface-coil MR imaging. *AJR Am J Roentgenol* 151:181–187, 1988.

Stiskal MA, Neuhold A, Szolar DH, et al: Rheumatoid arthritis of the craniocervical region by MR imaging: Detection and characterization. *AJR Am J Roentgenol* 165:585–592, 1995.

Cross-Reference

Neuroradiology: THE REQUISITES, p 501.

Comment

The T1-weighted sagittal image demonstrates a soft tissue mass with uniform, intermediate signal intensity extending from the anterior arch of C1 to the middle of the spinal canal. The upper portion of the odontoid process appears to be replaced by the mass, and cord compression is present at the cervicomedullary junction. The differential diagnosis includes primary bone tumor, chordoma, metastasis, plasmacytoma, lymphoma, or possibly meningioma, versus an inflammatory process such as pannus in a patient with rheumatoid arthritis or ankylosing spondylitis. The nasopharynx appears normal.

Pannus is defined as an inflammatory exudate overlying the lining layer of synovial cells on the inside of a joint; however, histologic findings in rheumatoid patients with inflamed synovium may vary from a fibrinous fluid collection in the joint space, to granulation tissue with abundant vessels, angioblasts, inflammatory cells, and soft tissue edema, to dense fibrous tissue without proliferating vessels or edema. Contrast-enhanced T1-weighted images of the craniocervical region may differentiate these variations, which have been categorized into four groups on the basis of their enhancement patterns: joint effusion, hypervascular pannus, hypovascular pannus, and fibrous pannus. These patterns have been detected even when plain radiographic studies are negative. Pannus is most commonly found in a retrodental location, which is the predominant location in this case. The synovial cell–lined articular capsules and bursae that may exhibit pannus formation are peridental-predental (C1–dens articulation), retrodental (transverse ligament–dens bursa), supradental (bursa), and zygapophyseal (facet joints) in location. Thickening of the ligaments and dura may also contribute to the appearance of a soft tissue mass.

Posterior subluxation, which is the least common of the five types of subluxation, is associated with an eroded odontoid. Vertical subluxation is also known as cranial settling and pseudobasilar invagination.

Notes

Syringohydromyelia, Postinflammatory

1. The second image was acquired 5 hours after the first one.

2. Increased CSF pressure, perhaps transient or periodic, forces CSF into the cord along the Virchow-Robin spaces.

3. Intramedullary elongated cystic regions lined by ependymal cells (hydromyelia) or glial cells (syringomyelia).

4. Hydromyelia.

Reference

Madsen PW III, Green BA, Bowen BC: Syringomyelia. In: Herkowitz HN, Garfin SR, Balderston RA, Eismont FJ, Bell GR, Wiesel SW, Eds: *Rothman-Simeone The Spine,* fourth edition. Philadelphia, WB Saunders, 1999, pp 1431–1459.

Cross-Reference

Neuroradiology: THE REQUISITES, pp 276, 484–485.

Comment

The axial CT images were obtained from the midthoracic spine after myelography. The first image was obtained 1 hour after the introduction of water-soluble contrast into the thecal sac via lumbar puncture. The cord is not grossly enlarged, and contrast fills the subarachnoid space. The second image was obtained 5 hours later, and now the contrast material has migrated into the cord and is filling a cavity that by comparison with the first image is a few millimeters smaller in diameter than the cord itself. Before the advent of MR imaging, postmyelography CT with early and delayed (4 to 6 hours) imaging was routinely used to determine whether an intramedullary cystic cavity was present. Unfortunately, not all intramedullary cysts demonstrate contrast accumulation on delayed images.

Several theories have been proposed regarding the development of intramedullary cystic cavities. Some theories invoke transmission of CSF pulsations into the central canal via the obex, as has been suggested in patients with Chiari I malformation. Others postulate a mechanism in which elevated CSF pressure—say, as a result of arachnoidal adhesions blocking the normal cranial flow of CSF around the cord—forces CSF into the cord along the Virchow-Robin spaces. In the latter theory, small collections of CSF coalesce to form larger syrinx cavities that may or may not communicate with the central canal. Syringomyelia refers to a central or eccentric, glial cell–lined, longitudinally oriented CSF-filled cavity, whereas hydromyelia refers to dilatation of the ependymal cell–lined central canal by CSF. Because the cyst lining cannot be identified on CT or MR imaging studies, the combined term *syringohydromyelia*, or simply "syrinx cavity," is used when describing these lesions.

Notes

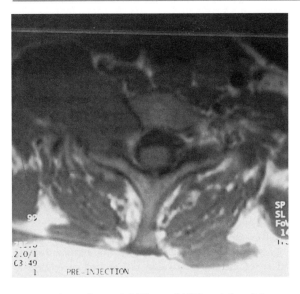
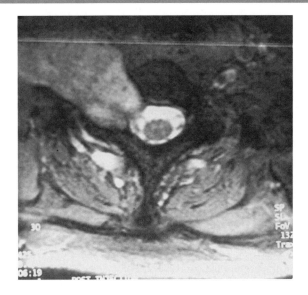

1. Based on the axial T1- and T2*-weighted images at C6-7, how do you explain the clinical findings of right brachial plexopathy involving the middle trunk?

2. Why is this disease unlikely to be lymphoma or metastasis?

3. Which muscle is displaced the most by this mass?

4. If this were a nerve sheath tumor, what additional imaging information would aid in the diagnosis?

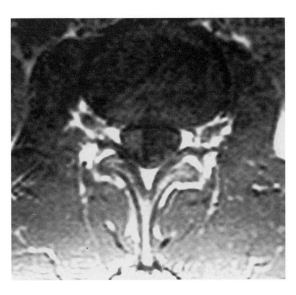
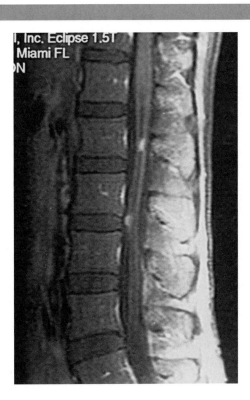

1. What intradural tumor typically involves the dorsal roots?

2. Based on the findings on the T1-weighted axial and postcontrast, fat-saturated sagittal images, would you recommend CT myelography, brain CT, brain MR imaging, or MR myelography as the next study?

3. List three "granulomatous diseases" that may produce pachymeningitis.

4. How often do these diseases coexist?

CASE 34

Extradural Schwannoma, Cervical

1. The mass involves the right C7 nerve. Its ventral ramus contributes to the plexus as the C7 root, which becomes the middle trunk.

2. The widened right neural foramen implies a chronic condition rather than an aggressive malignancy.

3. Anterior scalene.

4. If this lesion is solitary, it is almost certainly a schwannoma.

References

Lot G, George B: Cervical neuromas with extradural components: Surgical management in a series of 57 patients. *Neurosurgery* 41:813-820, 1997.

Mautner VF, Tatagiba M, Lindenau M, et al: Spinal tumors in patients with neurofibromatosis type 2: MR imaging study of frequency, multiplicity, and variety. *AJR Am J Roentgenol* 165:951-955, 1995.

Cross-Reference

Neuroradiology: THE REQUISITES, pp 489-490.

Comment

The axial images reveal a well-marginated extradural mass with a prolonged T2 relaxation time extending from the right C6-7 neural foramen to the paraspinal region. An important feature that could be confirmed with a CT scan is the apparently smooth widening of the neural foramen. This finding implies a chronic process favoring a benign neoplasm such as a nerve sheath tumor, hypertrophic neuropathy such as that of Dejerine-Sottas, or a complex meningeal cyst. By carefully tracking the lesion laterally, one may find that it courses between the anterior and middle scalene muscles, as expected for a neural lesion involving the roots of the brachial plexus. Although it is impossible to differientiate schwannoma from neurofibroma by imaging, solitary nerve sheath tumors in the spine are almost always schwannomas. These masses occur in patients without neurofibromatosis (as in this case) or in patients with neurofibromatosis type 2 (often in association with meningiomas and/or ependymomas). When a schwannoma reaches the size of the lesion in this case, it is common to find associated hemorrhage, cyst formation, and/or fatty degeneration, all of which result in heterogeneous signal intensity and enhancement. Lesions with both intradural and extradural components are usually narrowed at the neural foramen, resulting in a "dumbbell" appearance.

Notes

CASE 35

Sarcoidosis, Cauda Equina

1. Nerve sheath tumor (schwannoma/neurofibroma).

2. Brain MR imaging.

3. Sarcoidosis, tuberculosis, and fungal infection.

4. Patients with sarcoidosis have an increased incidence of tuberculosis (2% to 5%), as well as of fungal infections—*Aspergillus* mycetomas, candidiasis, and cryptococcosis.

References

Christoforidis GA, Spickler EM, Recio MV, Mehta BM: MR of CNS sarcoidosis: Correlation of imaging features to clinical symptoms and response to treatment. *AJNR Am J Neuroradiol* 20:655-669, 1999.

Lexa FJ, Grossman RI: MR of sarcoidosis in the head and spine: Spectrum of manifestations and radiographic response to steroid therapy. *AJNR Am J Neuroradiol* 15:973-982, 1994.

Cross-Reference

Neuroradiology: THE REQUISITES, p 480.

Comment

The precontrast axial and postcontrast, fat-saturated sagittal images demonstrate clumping of nerve roots, as well as smooth and nodular enhancement of the cauda equina. These findings are consistent with leptomeningeal disease, for which the differential diagnosis includes drop metastases from cord or brain tumors (e.g., glioblastoma multiforme, ependymoma, medulloblastoma), lymphoma, melanoma, carcinomatous meningitis (e.g., breast, lung, primary neoplasms), and infectious/inflammatory disorders, especially those that incite a granulomatous response in the host tissue. The next imaging study should be MR imaging with and without contrast enhancement of the remainder of the neural axis (brain and spine) to look for clues regarding the source of the lumbar leptomeningeal lesions. Myelographic studies would not add to the information already available from MR imaging with and without intravenous contrast.

Neurosarcoidosis has a variety of manifestations, including spinal cord masses and leptomeningitis with cauda equina syndrome and/or lumbosacral nerve root masses in the spine. In one study of 34 patients with a clinical diagnosis of neurosarcoidosis, 8 (24%) had spinal cord and nerve root involvement on MR imaging. The majority (7 of 8) were men, despite the fact that sarcoidosis more frequently affects females. In the brain the most common abnormal MR imaging finding is leptomeningeal and parenchymal enhancement in the region of the chiasm, floor of the third ventricle, and infundibulum, as well as white matter hyperintensities on T2-weighted images.

Notes

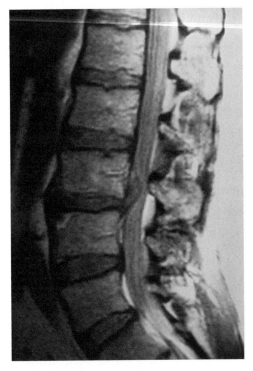 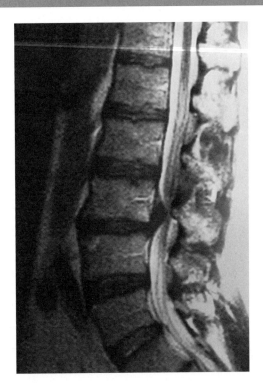

1. Approximately 90% of lumbar disk herniations involve which two levels: L3-4 and L4-5, or L4-5 and L5-S1?

2. One commonly used approach for characterizing disk herniation on MR imaging studies recognizes three descriptive types. Name them.

3. Which type corresponds to the findings on the proton-density-weighted and T2-weighted images shown here?

4. What reasons have been given to justify this approach?

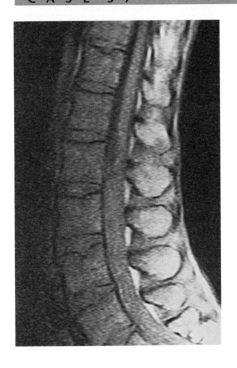

1. Name three conditions that may produce the intraspinal abnormality shown on this T1-weighted image.

2. What additional finding should be considered when formulating a differential diagnosis?

3. What are the major signs and symptoms of the clinical syndrome that this adult patient is likely to have?

4. What is the imaging study of choice to optimally characterize the abnormality?

C A S E 3 6

Disk Herniation (Extrusion), Lumbar

1. L4-5 and L5-S1.

2. Protrusion, extrusion, and sequestration.

3. Extrusion.

4. (1) Extrusion and sequestration may require a more extensive surgical approach than protrusion, (2) they are a contraindication to percutaneous diskectomy, and (3) such categorization may be helpful in differentiating asymptomatic from symptomatic disks.

References

Brant-Zawadzki MN, Jensen MC, Obuchowski N, Ross JS, Modic MT: Interobserver and intraobserver variability in interpretation of lumbar disc abnormalities. A comparison of two nomenclatures. *Spine* 20:1257–1263, 1995.

Jensen MC, Brant-Zawadzki MN, Obuchowski N, Modic MT, Malkasian D, Ross JS: Magnetic resonance imaging of the lumbar spine in people without back pain. *N Engl J Med* 331:69–73, 1994.

Modic MT: Degenerative disorders of the spine. In: Modic MT, Masaryk TJ, Ross JS, Eds: *Magnetic Resonance Imaging of the Spine.* Chicago, Year Book, 1989, pp 75–119.

Cross-Reference

Neuroradiology: THE REQUISITES, pp 461–463.

Comment

The sagittal images show disk herniation (extrusion) at the L3-4 interspace with cephalic extension posterior to the L3 body (the extension beyond the interspace was focal on axial images). The portion of disk within the canal appears to be (1) connected by a slightly thinner pedicle to the portion of disk remaining in the L3-4 interspace and (2) contained posteriorly by a curvilinear rim of low signal intensity representing an intact posterior longitudinal ligament (inseparable from the low signal of dura). This defect is sometimes called a subligamentous herniation. The herniated portion may or may not have high signal intensity on T2-weighted images as compared with the portion in the interspace.

The generally accepted nomenclature for degenerative disk pathology is as follows: disks extending beyond the interspace are categorized as bulging (symmetric, circumferential extension), protruded (asymmetric or symmetric, focal extension, with a roughly conical shape pointing posteriorly and residual low–signal intensity annular fibers), or extruded (as described earlier for this case, without or with caudal or cephalic extension but with complete rupture of anular fibers). Protruded or extruded disks are herniated disks. A sequestered disk is an extruded disk with a dissociated fragment ("free fragment"). Differentiation of protrusion from extrusion may be of clinical significance: a blinded study of asymptomatic subjects found that 52% had a disk bulge and 27% had a protrusion, whereas only 1% had an extrusion.

Notes

C A S E 3 7

Leptomeningeal Carcinomatosis

1. Leptomeningeal metastases (carcinomatosis), lymphoma, and filum/cauda ependymoma.

2. Most of the vertebral bodies are relatively hypointense, which may result from fatty marrow replacement secondary to hematopoietic malignancy or certain chemotherapy regimens.

3. Cauda equina syndrome: (1) buttock or leg pain, lower extremity weakness, and loss of bladder and rectal sphincter control; (2) loss of sensation in the saddle area, the posterior aspect of each thigh, and the lateral aspect of each foot; and (3) diminished deep tendon reflexes.

4. Contrast-enhanced T1-weighted MR imaging with fat suppression.

Reference

Gomori JM, Heching N, Siegal T: Leptomeningeal metastases: Evaluation by gadolinium enhanced spinal magnetic resonance imaging. *J Neurooncol* 36:55–60, 1998.

Cross-Reference

Neuroradiology: THE REQUISITES, pp 487–488.

Comment

On this sagittal T1-weighted image, the normal low signal intensity of CSF is seen only above the level of L2. Below this level, a "mass" that is isointense relative to cord fills the canal. Sheet-like, linear, or nodular enhancement of this "mass" on gadolinium-enhanced T1-weighted images favors leptomeningeal metastatic disease or lymphoma. The additional finding of diffuse hypointensity of the vertebral bodies, as compared with the disk spaces, supports a diagnosis of lymphoma or other hematopoietic malignancy. Widespread metastatic carcinoma, however, is not excluded from the differential diagnosis, and the possibility of time-dependent, treatment-related marrow changes must be considered. Filum ependymoma appears as an elongated, circumscribed mass with marked homogeneous or heterogeneous enhancement. An ependymoma of this size might have produced bony erosion with scalloping of the posterior margin of one or more lumbar vertebrae. A nerve sheath tumor or meningioma of such size is extremely rare. Furthermore, these tumors would not account for the hypointense vertebral bodies.

Notes

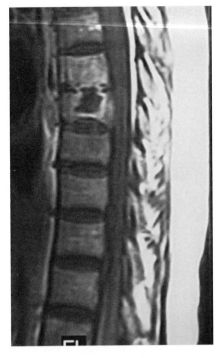
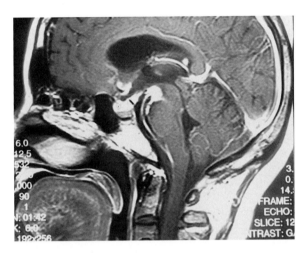

1. List four types of inflammatory lesions shown on the postcontrast T1-weighted sagittal images of the thoracolumbar spine and brain.

2. Do the findings favor a pyogenic or a granulomatous disease?

3. What is the primary mechanism producing the findings?

4. What coexisting condition would you expect to find in this 45-year-old woman?

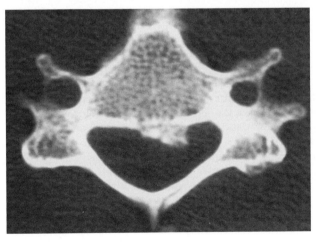
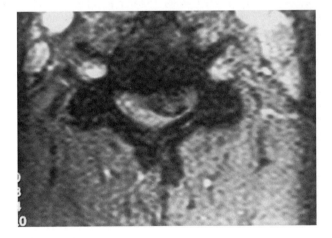

1. What magnetic property of tissues could explain the apparent discrepancy in size of this C5 osteophyte on the gradient-recalled-echo (GRE) MR image versus the CT image?

2. How would you modify the GRE sequence parameters to lessen the discrepancy?

3. What pulse sequence would you suggest as an alternative to the GRE sequence to lessen the discrepancy?

4. Name three other lesions that may produce the findings shown on the CT and MR images.

Craniospinal Tuberculosis

1. Vertebral osteomyelitis, diskitis, meningitis, and cerebral (subependymal) granuloma.

2. Granulomatous disease.

3. Hematogenous spread of mycobacteria via the arteries and arterioles to the vertebral end-plates, meninges, and brain parenchyma.

4. Acquired immunodeficiency syndrome (AIDS).

References

Sharif HS, Morgan JL, al Shahed MS, al Thagafi MY: Role of CT and MR imaging in the management of tuberculous spondylitis. *Radiol Clin North Am* 33:787-804, 1995.

Whiteman MLH, Bowen BC, Post MJD, Pell MD: Intracranial infection. In: Atlas SW, Ed: *Magnetic Resonance Imaging of the Brain and Spine,* second edition. Philadelphia, Lippincott-Raven, 1996, pp 707-772.

Cross-Reference
Neuroradiology: THE REQUISITES, pp 478-479.

Comment

The postcontrast images demonstrate a constellation of vertebral, leptomeningeal, and brain parenchymal features that favor granulomatous infection, with pyogenic infection, metastatic disease, and lymphoma being less likely. On the thoracolumbar image, a destructive lesion within T8 extends to the T7-8 disk space and exhibits ring enhancement. Axial images (not shown) indicated epidural extension in the left side of the canal, as well as paraspinal involvement. Leptomeningeal enhancement of the cauda equina is evident at the inferior margin of the spine image. On the brain image, striking enhancement is noted along meningeal surfaces in the prepontine cistern, interpeduncular cistern, suprasellar cistern, and cistern of the lamina terminalis. An enhancing nodule is seen anterior to the splenium in the velum interpositum.

It can be difficult to distinguish tuberculous from pyogenic osteomyelitis/diskitis. Tuberculous osteomyelitis, which typically affects the lower thoracic spine, is favored in conditions with relatively limited involvement of the disk space in comparison with the vertebral body. In particular, rim enhancement around an intraosseous abscess on postcontrast T1-weighted images (as in this case) is a characteristic of tuberculosis (TB) that is only occasionally demonstrated in other spinal infections. When compared with *Brucella* or pyogenic osteomyelitis, tuberculous osteomyelitis is more likely to have prominent paraspinal and epidural masses and to spare the posterior elements. Leptomeningeal enhancement involving the intracranial basal cisterns and the cauda equina is consistent with tuberculous meningitis and further supports a diagnosis of systemic TB with hematogenous spread to the brain and spine. TB is estimated to be up to 500 times more common in patients with AIDS than in HIV-negative individuals. CNS tuberculosis occurs in 2% to 5% of patients with TB and in 10% of those with AIDS-associated TB.

Notes

Magnetic Susceptibility Effects (Blooming Artifact)

1. Magnetic susceptibility.

2. Shorten the echo time (TE) and decrease the voxel size.

3. T2-weighted fast-spin-echo sequence.

4. Ossification of the posterior longitudinal ligament (OPLL), calcified herniated disk (migrated), and meningioma.

Reference

Tien RD, Buxton RB, Schwaighofer BW, Chu PK: Quantitation of structural distortion of the cervical neural foramina in gradient-echo MR imaging. *J Magn Reson Imaging* 1:683-687, 1991.

Cross-Reference
Neuroradiology: THE REQUISITES, pp 8-9.

Comment

On the axial GRE image (5-mm-thick slice), the hypointense area in the left side of the canal is much larger than the size of the osteophyte. Most of this additional hypointensity is due to susceptibility effects ("blooming artifact"), whereas a portion represents cord that is displaced to the right. Inside the hypointense area is a slightly hyperintense region that may be attributed to partial volume averaging with adjacent CSF signal. A thin hyperintense band, primarily representing CSF signal, is seen at the posterior margin of the hypointense area.

Transverse relaxation of proton spins has three components: T2 from spin-spin relaxation (an intrinsic tissue property), T2′ from main field inhomogeneity, and T2″ from susceptibility effects. The effective transverse relaxation rate, $1/T2^*$, is given by the equation

$$1/T2^* = 1/T2 + 1/T2' + 1/T2''$$

($T2^*$ is called the effective transverse relaxation time; rate = 1/time). For spin-echo sequences the 180° refocusing pulse rephases both the T2′ and T2″ so that only the T2 relaxation time varies from tissue to tissue, producing image contrast (a T2-weighted image). GRE sequences use a magnetic field gradient pulse (usually the read gradient) to refocus the spins. The gradient pulse does not rephase the T2′ and T2″ components, so all three components determine image contrast (a T2*-weighted image). In tissue regions where susceptibility effects are considerable, T2″ is very short, and $1/T2''$ determines $1/T2^*$. Thus, $T2^*$ is shortened, and the region appears more hypointense on a GRE image than on a spin-echo image.

Magnetic susceptibility is a property of tissue that measures how much a tissue alters the external, applied magnetic field. When two adjacent tissues, such as the bone (osteophyte) and CSF in this case, have very different susceptibilities, marked distortion of the local magnetic field occurs and extends over a relatively long distance. The distortion causes dephasing of the proton spins and is responsible for the T2″ and T2* shortening and the consequent signal loss encompassing the left half of the spinal canal.

Notes

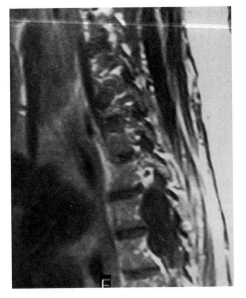
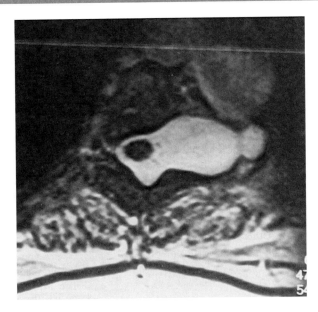

1. The abnormality shown on the postcontrast T1-weighted parasagittal image and on the T2*-weighted GRE (gradient-recalled-echo) axial image is associated with which of the phakomatoses?

2. What symptoms, if any, result from the abnormality?

3. What percentage of patients with this abnormality have bilateral lesions?

4. What is Lehman's syndrome?

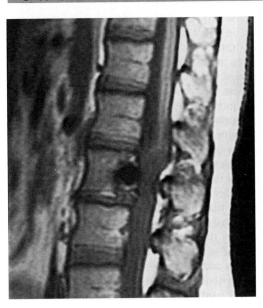
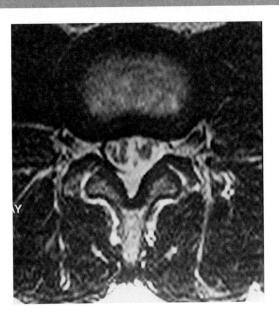

1. Based on the T1-weighted sagittal and the T2-weighted fast-spin-echo axial (L3-4 level) images, what feature may explain the progressive myeloradiculopathy in this 35-year-old man?

2. What surgical procedure may be helpful in halting the progressive clinical deficits?

3. Are the majority of bullet fragments strongly ferromagnetic?

4. In a patient with a metallic foreign body, does a safe MR imaging examination mean that a repeat MR study will be safe for the patient?

Metastatic Melanoma, Epidural and Intradural

1. Metastatic disease. The differential diagnosis includes lymphoma and leukemia.

2. Because the leptomeningeal lesions may be the result of CSF seeding from a brain parenchymal metastasis rather than the result of hematogenous dissemination.

3. Neurofibromatosis type 1.

4. Late.

Reference

Gokaslan ZL, Aladag MA, Ellerhorst JA: Melanoma metastatic to the spine: A review of 133 cases. *Melanoma Res* 10:78–80, 2000.

Cross-Reference

Neuroradiology: THE REQUISITES, pp 488, 491.

Comment

The axial image at T4 provides evidence of an epidural and paraspinal enhancing mass with involvement of the left fourth rib, transverse process, and costovertebral area. From the sagittal and axial (T12 level) images, vertebral and intradural (leptomeningeal) lesions are evident. The combination of extraspinal and intraspinal lesions suggests metastatic disease or lymphoma, and the presence of a paraspinal thoracic mass would seem to favor a primary lung carcinoma. Melanoma metastasizes widely and, along with lung and breast cancer, is one of the most common causes of leptomeningeal "carcinomatosis." Leptomeningeal deposits of melanoma metastases may result from hematogenous dissemination or from CSF seeding of a brain metastasis, which this patient had. Although primary brain tumors may also seed the spinal leptomeninges via the subarachnoid space ("drop mets"), they rarely cause extradural and vertebral metastases and are thus virtually excluded from the differential diagnosis in this case. As can be seen from the fat-saturated postcontrast T1-weighted image, vertebral body metastases are present at several upper thoracic levels, without vertebral collapse. Vertebral metastases occur relatively late in the course of metastatic melanoma (cutaneous, ocular, or mucosal origin) and herald a poor prognosis because the median survival for these patients is about 4 months.

Notes

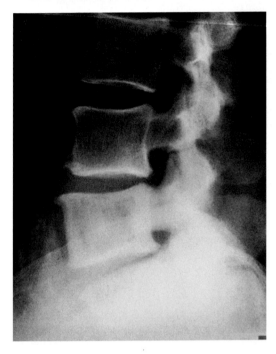
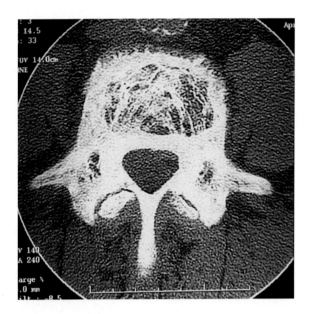

1. List four causes of the neurologic symptoms (e.g., radiculopathy, cauda equina syndrome, or myelopathy) that may occur as a result of the disease shown here involving only L5.

2. List five causes of a dense, sclerotic vertebra.

3. What is the most common complication of this disease, and does it occur early or late in the disease process?

4. Is L4 or L5 more likely to be the site of lytic metastasis in the future?

Paget's Disease

1. Vertebral enlargement (as illustrated in this case) producing spinal stenosis, ossification of extradural structures also producing spinal stenosis, pathologic vertebral fracture, and facet arthropathy.

2. Osteoblastic metastasis, Paget's disease, lymphoma, myelosclerosis (myeloid metaplasia), and fracture (compression or healing).

3. Pathologic fracture occurs during the early osteolytic phase of Paget's disease.

4. L5, because metastases selectively involve pagetic bone—presumably because of its hypervascularity.

Reference

Poncelet A: The neurologic complications of Paget's disease. *J Bone Miner Res* 14(suppl 2):88–91, 1999.

Cross-Reference

Neuroradiology: THE REQUISITES, p 495.

Comment

The lateral view of the lumbar spine in this 61-year-old man demonstrates a hyperdense, enlarged (anterior-posterior direction) L5 vertebral body with a thickened cortex that forms a "picture frame" around the body, as well as apparent thickening of the pedicles. The thickened cortex and the coarse trabeculation of cancellous bone are evident on the CT image, as is enlargement of the posterior elements without significant spinal stenosis. The bone remodeling has also affected the facet joints, which show narrowing of the joint spaces and hypertrophic changes of the facets, consistent with a moderate pagetic facet arthropathy.

Paget's disease, a condition of unknown etiology, generally occurs after the age of 50 years. Radiographically, three phases may be seen: osteolytic (early, active), mixed (intermediate), and osteoblastic (late, inactive). In this case, L5 has features of both mixed and osteoblastic phases (all three phases may coexist in the same bone), with bone remodeling producing thickened cortex and coarse trabeculation of the cancellous bone on the axial CT image. When a more uniform increase in bone density is noted, the possibility of lymphoma or metastatic prostate cancer should be considered; however, these conditions are unlikely to cause expansion of the vertebra. Monostotic disease may be mistaken for fibrous dysplasia.

Enlargement of the vertebral body and/or the neural arch may produce spinal stenosis, which reportedly occurs in about 80% of symptomatic (pain with or without neurologic symptoms) patients and 20% of asymptomatic patients. Pagetic facet arthropathy also reportedly occurs in about 80% of symptomatic patients. Compression fractures of involved vertebral bodies are usually asymptomatic but occasionally lead to neurologic symptoms. Vascular mechanisms have also been proposed to account for the symptoms, including (1) a steal of blood flow to the cord and nerve roots by nearby hypermetabolic pagetic bone and (2) compression of the anterior spinal artery by expanded bone.

Primary malignant bone tumors are 20 times more likely to develop in individuals with Paget's disease than in age-matched controls. Osteosarcoma is the most common histologic type, followed by fibrosarcoma and chondrosarcoma. Sarcomatous transformation is heralded by the development of a lytic lesion, sometimes with cortical breakthrough, pathologic fracture, and/or a soft tissue mass. The differential diagnosis includes lytic or blastic metastases (e.g., breast, prostate, or kidney primary sites) to pagetic bone, which have been reported to occur selectively.

Notes

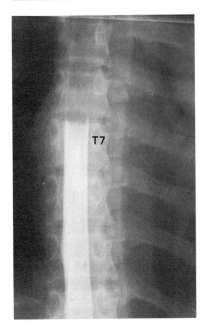

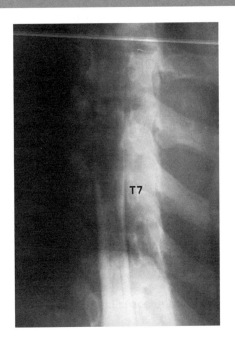

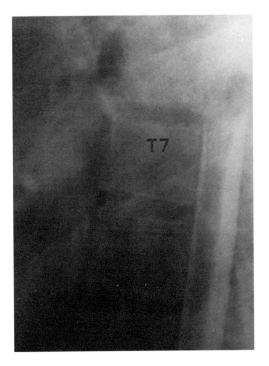

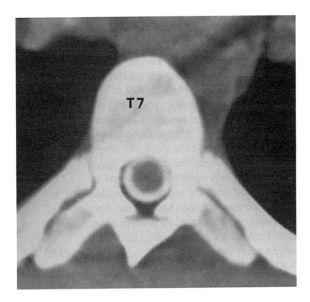

1. How are spinal tumors classified with regard to myelographic findings?

2. What is a "spinal block" or "spinal cord block"?

3. Give two examples of lumbar disk herniation that may not be detected by myelography.

4. What intradural lesions may be difficult to identify on MR imaging or CT but are often readily shown on myelography?

Sagittal, Epidural Midline Septum

1. Anatomically, the anterior epidural space is defined as the region between the theca and the posterior surface of the vertebral bodies. The PLL, areolar connective tissue, fat, and a venous network are located within this region.

2. Anulus fibrosus at the level of the disk space, sagittal septum posterior to the vertebral body, and lateral membrane.

3. False. It is separated by the lateral membrane, which inserts on the lateral wall of the spinal canal.

4. Lumbar. The cervical epidural space contains predominantly blood vessels and perivascular connective tissue.

Reference

Schellinger D, Manz HJ, Vidic B, et al: Disk fragment migration. *Radiology* 175:831–836, 1990.

Cross-Reference

Neuroradiology: THE REQUISITES, pp 461–463.

Comment

As shown on this axial image at the level of the L4 pedicles, a predominantly fat-filled space is located between the posterior surface of the vertebral body and the thecal sac. The hypointense line at the margin of the thecal sac represents the anterior theca and PLL. Perpendicular to this line is a sagittally oriented hypointense band in the midline—the "sagittal midline septum"—which consists of lamellae of compact collagen. At its anterior extent the septum merges with another hypointense line, which is the periosteum of the vertebral body. The midline septum thus spans the anterior epidural space from the PLL to the periosteum and divides the space into two compartments. The superior and inferior margins of these compartments are formed by the insertion of the PLL into the anulus fibrosus (i.e., no midline septum is opposite the disk space). The lateral margins are formed by a delicate membrane (not seen here) that stretches laterally from the free edge of the PLL to the lateral wall of the canal. The effect of the midline septum is to direct migrated and sequestered disk fragments into either the left- or right-sided compartment.

Notes

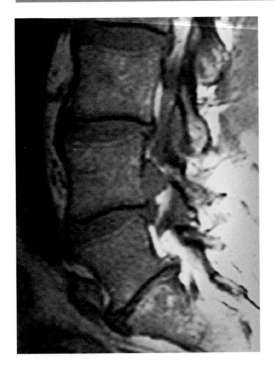

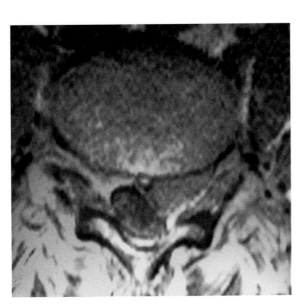

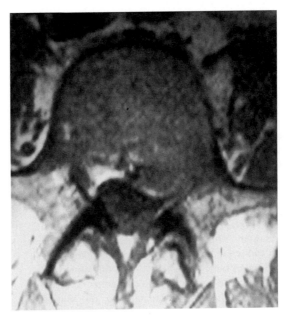

1. You are shown left parasagittal and axial T1-weighted images (without intravenous contrast). The axial images were obtained at the level of the L4-5 disk space (left image) and at the level of the L4 pedicles (right image). Why is the anterior epidural mass confined to the left side of the midline at the level of the pedicles?

2. Why is the term *herniated disk* preferred to *herniated nucleus pulposus*?

3. Can a disk have more than one herniation?

4. Give an example of two herniations by the same disk.

Herniated Disk Constrained by Midline Septum

1. The mass, which is a herniated (extruded) disk with superior migration, is constrained to the left anterior epidural compartment by the sagittal midline septum. Epidural fat outlines the posterior margin of the migrated disk in the axial image at the level of the L4 pedicles.

2. Because tissues other than the nucleus are common components of displaced disk material. These tissues include cartilage, fragmented apophyseal bone, and fragmented anulus.

3. Yes.

4. Herniation through an anular fissure or tear into the anterior epidural space (as shown here), and herniation through a break in an adjacent vertebral body end-plate (intravertebral herniation, or Schmorl's node).

References

Fardon DF, Milette PC: Nomenclature and classification of lumbar disc pathology: recommendations of the combined task forces of the north american spine society, american society of spine radiology, and american society of neuroradiology. *Spine* 26:E93–E113, 2001.

Schellinger D, Manz HJ, Vidic B, et al: Disk fragment migration. *Radiology* 175:831–836, 1990.

Cross-Reference

Neuroradiology: THE REQUISITES, pp 461–463.

Comment

Schellinger and colleagues have reported that when herniated disks (extruded disks, with or without sequestration) migrate either superiorly or inferiorly, the migrated component is found predominantly in either the left or right half of the anterior epidural space in 94% of cases. The migrated component straddles the midline in only 6% of cases. Based on studies of cadaver specimens, the authors concluded that the anterior epidural space opposite the vertebral body is divided into a left and a right compartment by a collagenous, sagittal midline septum (adherent to the posterior longitudinal ligament and the vertebral body periosteum). The migrating disk is thus directed into and loosely constrained to either compartment. If the disk is pushed across the midline, the leading edge is smoothly capped by the bowed and potentially detachable midline septum. Schellinger and associates also found no preferred direction of migration (42% superior, 40% inferior, and 18% bidirectional), and moreover, no consensus on migration direction can be found in the literature.

Currently, a concerted effort is being made by spine radiologists, neurologists, surgeons, and other interested medical professionals to develop a standardized nomenclature and classification system for lumbar disk pathology. In this nomenclature herniated disks may take the form of protrusions or extrusions. A sequestration is a specific form of extrusion in which the displaced disk material has completely lost all continuity with the parent disk. To describe the location of a herniated disk in the axial (horizontal) plane, several terms referring to "anatomic zones" have been proposed. Moving from a central to a lateral direction for a left-sided herniated disk, the location would be identified as "central," "left central," "left subarticular," "left foraminal," or "left extraforaminal" (synonymous with "far lateral"). As in this example, a large herniated disk may span more than one zone. In the sagittal (craniocaudal) plane, anatomic zones, which can be used to describe the extent of migration, are loosely defined as the "disk level," the "infrapedicular level," the "pedicular level," and the "suprapedicular level." In this case the disk has migrated to the pedicular level.

Notes

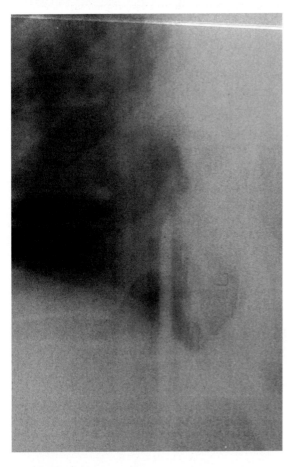

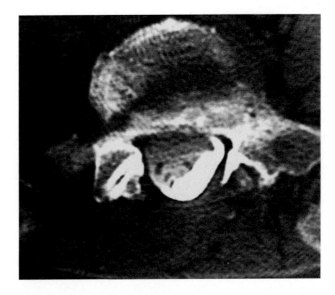

1. What is wrong with the myelogram and postmyelogram CT scan shown here?

2. How might this problem be avoided?

3. To delineate the extent of a myelographic "spinal block," it may be necessary to inject contrast via a cervical (C1-2) puncture and a lumbar puncture. Which puncture should be done first?

4. What is the most important principle to remember when interpreting myelograms?

Subdural Injection of Contrast

1. A relatively large amount of contrast material is located in the subdural space.

2. When contrast is injected after lumbar puncture, look for free flow of contrast away from the needle tip and gradual visualization of the roots of the cauda equina.

3. Lumbar puncture.

4. All lesions must be viewed in at least two planes.

Reference

Benson JE, Hon JS: Examination of the spine: Myelography. In: Taveras JM, Ferrucci JT, Eds: *Radiology, Diagnosis-Imaging-Intervention,* Vol 3. Philadelphia, JB Lippincott, 1988, pp 7–11.

Cross-Reference

Neuroradiology: THE REQUISITES, pp 455–457.

Comment

The lateral radiograph, obtained with the patient in the prone position, shows a dense collection of contrast with a tapered contour and sharp leading edge that has tracked along the posterior aspect of the spinal canal from the lumbar to the lower thoracic region (leading edge is at the T9-10 level). This subdural collection has resulted from a lumbar puncture. Anterior to the subdural collection, less dense contrast is present in the subarachnoid space and is partially outlining the spinal cord. The appearance of a subdural collection on CT is shown in the second image (different patient, L5-S1 level). Note the peripheral, posterior-lateral location of the collection in the thecal sac, as well as the inward displacement of the cauda equina nerve roots. Contrast material is also present in the subarachnoid space and is causing faintly increased density of the CSF surrounding the nerve roots.

Each of these patients has actually had a "mixed injection" (subdural plus subarachnoid space) of contrast material via lumbar puncture. To avoid this situation, one must observe the flow and accumulation of contrast during injection. Contrast should not collect at the tip of the spinal needle; instead, it should disperse freely and cause a gradual increase in density in the canal around the nerve roots, which appear as "filling defects." If the roots are not seen and contrast has collected posteriorly in the canal on a lateral radiograph (as shown here), suspect a predominantly subdural injection. Repositioning of the needle is warranted before further injection of contrast. In cases of severe arachnoiditis, the filling defects of individual nerve roots may not be seen, even though contrast has been instilled in the subarachnoid space.

In a patient with myelopathy and suspected spinal block, injection of contrast above and below the block may be necessary to determine its extent. If the cervical puncture is done first, contrast is instilled in the cervical region above the block. When the lumbar puncture is subsequently done, it is usually necessary to put the patient in a head-down position for contrast to flow to the lower edge of the block. By putting the patient head-down, however, the contrast above the block flows into the head, becomes diluted in the basal cisterns,

and may leave insufficient contrast to delineate the block. Thus, it is advantageous to do the lumbar puncture before the cervical puncture when both procedures are performed in a single examination.

Sometimes the need to perform two punctures can be avoided by doing a postmyelogram CT scan after the first puncture even though contrast material cannot be detected beyond the block on the myelogram. The high sensitivity of CT allows much lower concentrations of contrast material to be detected, so the extent of the obstructing mass can still be determined. Postmyelogram CT may also provide diagnostic information on intraspinal masses despite a mixed injection and decreased contrast material in the subarachnoid space.

Notes

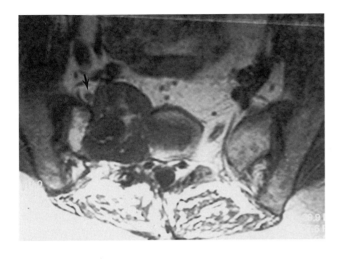
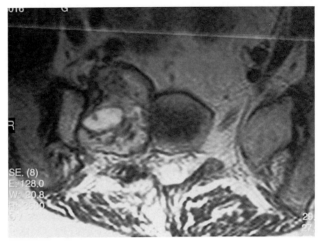
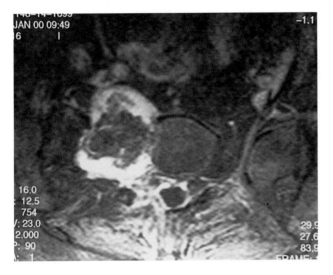

1. Is this mass more likely to be a malignant or a benign lesion? Why?

2. Name the three most common malignant tumors that "originate" in the sacrum (i.e., cause sacral destruction intrinsically).

3. Based on the T1-weighted, fast-spin-echo T2-weighted, and postcontrast fat-saturated T1-weighted images, how much of the sacral plexus is involved by the mass?

4. Biopsy of the tumor revealed a cellular neoplasm composed of short intersecting fascicles and whorls of uniform spindle cells lacking hyperchromasia and pleomorphism. The mitotic count was low, and strong, diffuse staining for S100 protein was observed. Your diagnosis?

Schwannoma, Sacral

1. Benign; it has smooth, rounded margins and does not invade the adjacent fat. CT scan would verify the apparent sclerotic rim of bone at the interface of the right sacral ala and the mass. Nevertheless, benign and malignant peripheral nerve sheath tumors may be indistinguishable, and biopsy is necessary for diagnosis.

2. Chordoma, chondrosarcoma, and metastatic lesions.

3. Based on these axial images, only the S1 ventral ramus is involved.

4. Schwannoma.

References

Dominguez J, Lobato RD, Ramos A, Rivas JJ, Gomez PA, Castro S: Giant intrasacral schwannomas: Report of six cases. *Acta Neurochir (Wien)* 139:954–959, 1997.

Lin PP, Horenstein MG, Healey JH: Sacral mass in a 56-year-old woman. *Clin Orthop* 344:333–337, 341–343, 1997.

Cross-Reference

Neuroradiology: THE REQUISITES, pp 489–490.

Comment

The precontrast and postcontrast MR images demonstrate an inhomogeneous mass with solid and cystic areas, apparent encapsulation, and nonaggressive features. The mass is primarily located within the right S1 neural foramen, in the expected location of the S1 nerve (note the normal left S1 nerve). The right lumbosacral trunk *(arrow)* and the intradural S2 nerve are separate from the mass in this 74-year-old woman, who previously had right hemilaminectomy and biopsy of the mass.

Spinal schwannomas are relatively uncommon, and less than 1% to 5% occur in the sacrum. Histologically, schwannomas are characterized by alternating Antoni A and Antoni B areas with cellular and hypocellular regions, respectively. They are encapsulated lesions that typically do not compromise nerve function but may cause paresthesias or pain from pressure. A variant of the conventional schwannoma is the cellular schwannoma, which is composed predominantly of Antoni A areas, lacks Verocay bodies, and is predominantly found in the retroperitoneum, pelvis, and paraspinal area of the mediastinum. Sacral schwannomas, often designated "giant" because of the enormous size that they may attain, destroy the sacrum and expand into the pelvis, spinal canal, and dorsal muscle and fat. The differential diagnosis for a sacral mass includes malignant and benign lesions. The MR features are not those of a malignant lesion, and the signal characteristics of the myxoid matrix found in chordoma and chondrosarcoma are lacking. Benign bone lesions such as giant cell tumor, aneurysmal bone cyst, and osteoblastoma occur infrequently in the sacrum, and the latter two typically involve posterior elements. Rarely, sacrococcygeal teratoma and myxopapillary ependymoma occur in the presacral area.

Notes

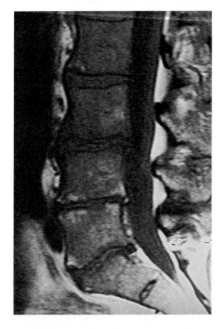 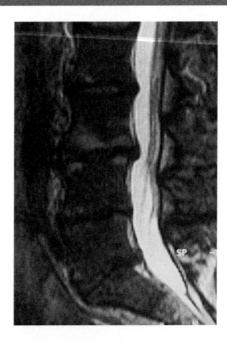

1. What are the three types of so-called end-plate changes?
2. Which types are present at levels L3-4 and L4-5 in this case?
3. Which type, if any, demonstrates postcontrast enhancement?
4. How might disk degeneration mask disk space infection on T1-weighted images?

Degenerative Changes in Vertebral Body Marrow ("End-Plate Changes")

1. Signal intensity on T1- and T2-weighted images: low and high (type I), respectively; high and intermediate/high (type II); and low and low (type III).

2. L3-4 = type I; L4-5 = type II.

3. Type I, which is characterized by enhancement of the vascularized fibrous tissue.

4. The low signal intensity within the vertebral marrow caused by infection may be masked by the high signal intensity associated with type II degenerative changes. T2-weighted images help clarify the diagnosis: high signal intensity within the disk space favors infection, whereas low signal intensity favors disk degeneration.

References

de Roos A, Kressel H, Spritzer C, Dalinka M: MR imaging of marrow changes adjacent to end plates in degenerative lumbar disk disease. *AJR Am J Roentgenol* 149:531–534, 1987.

Modic MT, Steinberg PM, Ross JS, Masaryk TJ, Carter JR: Degenerative disk disease: Assessment of changes in vertebral body marrow with MR imaging. *Radiology* 166:193–199, 1988.

Cross-Reference

Neuroradiology: THE REQUISITES, p 466.

Comment

The signal intensity within the vertebral body marrow adjacent to the end-plate at the level of a degenerated disk may be increased or decreased in comparison with normal marrow. The combination of signal intensity changes on T1- and T2-weighted images reflects the underlying histopathologic changes and has been categorized by Modic and others as type I, II, or III changes. For type I changes (low on T1-weighted and high on T2-weighted images), fibrovascular tissue replaces the hematopoietic and lipid elements of normal marrow. Type I changes may mimic the MR findings for vertebral osteomyelitis; however, osteomyelitis is usually accompanied by diskitis, which results in an abnormal configuration and high signal intensity of the intervertebral disk space. These disk space abnormalities differ from the usual observation of low signal intensity for the degenerated disk (as shown here at L3-4); however, some degenerated disks contain cystic areas that are bright on T2-weighted images and thus indistinguishable from early infection.

For type II changes (high on T1-weighted and intermediate/high on T2-weighted images), the lipid content of the marrow space is increased (i.e., more "yellow marrow") in comparison with normal. The signal intensity on T2-weighted images depends in part on the pulse sequence used—the fast-spin-echo sequence typically yields higher signal intensity than does the standard spin-echo sequence. Type I changes have been observed to convert to type II changes with time, whereas type II changes are relatively stable. Type III changes most likely represent areas of marrow replacement by dense woven bone because these changes correspond to areas of bony sclerosis on plain radiographs.

Notes

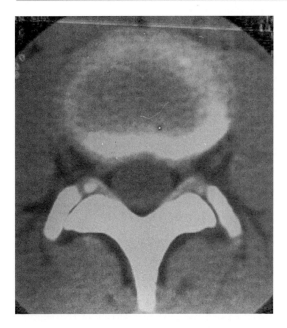

1. Name four entities that may account for the hyperdensity medial to the right superior articular process of L3.
2. As a normal variant, what is the most common location for this hyperdensity?
3. What separates it from the articular facet?
4. How frequently is it bilateral or multiple?

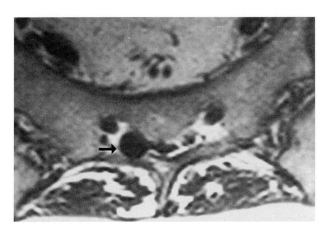
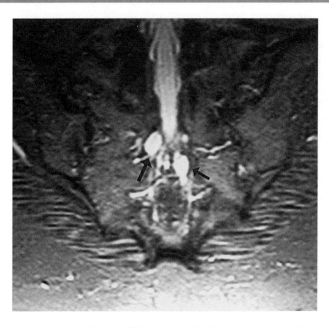

1. The sacral cysts, indicated by the *arrows* on the T1-weighted axial (left) and T2-weighted oblique coronal (right) images, typically arise from which spinal structures?
2. Are the cysts predominantly intradural or extradural?
3. Are they likely to contain only CSF?
4. Are they usually associated with enlargement of the anterior or the posterior (synonymous with ventral and dorsal, respectively, as used here) sacral foramina?

Unfused Ossicle*

1. Fracture fragment, facet spur or osteophyte, calcification of the ligamentum flavum, and accessory ossicle.

2. Inferior articular processes of L2 or L3.

3. A fluid-filled space contiguous with the facet joint.

4. In approximately 20% of cases.

Reference

Pech P, Haughton VM: CT appearance of unfused ossicles in the lumbar spine. *AJNR Am J Neuroradiol* 6:629–631, 1985.

Cross-Reference

Neuroradiology: THE REQUISITES, pp 449–451.

Comment

This well-corticated osseous density adjacent to the right superior articular process of L3 is presumably an unfused ossicle. It was detected incidentally on lumbar CT in a 17-year-old girl with no history of trauma. Unfused ossicles result from accessory ossification centers near the tips of the vertebral processes. The most common location is L2 or L3, as noted above. In anatomic sections, the space that separates the ossicle from the articular process is filled with fluid resembling synovial fluid. Although not yet described on MR imaging, this space may be identifiable by its hyperintensity on T2-weighted images and hypointensity on T1-weighted images.

The ossicle is located behind the ligamentum flavum and is often shown best on reformatted sagittal or coronal CT images. The incidence of lumbar unfused ossicles has been estimated at 0.5% to 1.5% in the general population based on early studies that relied on plain radiographs for detection of ossicles.

---

*Figure for Case 50 from Pech P, Haughton VM: CT appearance of unfused ossicles in the lumbar spine. *AJNR Am J Neuroradiol* 6:629–631, 1985.

Notes

Tarlov Cysts

1. Posterior nerve root sleeves.

2. Extradural.

3. No. Posterior nerve root fibers and/or ganglion cells are present in the cyst wall or bathed in CSF within the cyst.

4. Posterior (i.e., dorsal) sacral foramina, as suggested by the axial image.

Reference

Davis SW, Levy LM, LeBihan DJ, Rajan S, Schellinger D: Sacral meningeal cysts: Evaluation with MR imaging. *Radiology* 187:445–448, 1993.

Cross-Reference

Neuroradiology: THE REQUISITES, p 484.

Comment

On the axial image (S1-2 level), the right-sided cyst (*arrow*) is contiguous with the thecal sac and the S2 root and appears to have partially eroded the posterior surface of the sacrum. On the oblique coronal image (approximately parallel to the plane of the sacrum), the cyst (*large arrow*) is in the region of the right S2 nerve root, whereas a smaller cyst (*small arrow*) is in the region of the left S3 nerve root. These cysts are typical perineurial, or Tarlov, cysts. They are diverticula of the nerve root sheath and may or may not communicate with the spinal subarachnoid space. Davis and colleagues found that cysts that communicate with the subarachnoid space, based on the finding of flow-related signal loss in the cysts with the use of two-dimensional motion-sensitive MR pulse sequences, were clinically asymptomatic. Cysts that did not communicate, that is, did not show internal flow patterns, were symptomatic (sciatica).

In the system of Nabors and colleagues, Tarlov cysts are classified as type II spinal meningeal cysts based on their extradural location and the presence of nerve root fibers in the cysts. The presence of nerve root fibers is established by surgical examination and histopathologic review, not by MR imaging. Thus, on imaging, type II cysts may not be distinguishable from sacral type I cysts, which are also extradural in location and yet are diverticula of the meningeal sac that lack nerve root fibers. Type I cysts tend to have a pedicle, however, whereas type II cysts do not.

When considering sacral nerve roots, one must remember that the dorsal ganglion is located along the posterior (dorsal) root in the canal and that below the ganglion, the posterior root (or ramus) is a peripheral nerve that exits the sacrum through a posterior foramen. The perineurium and endoneurium of the exiting nerve are peripheral extensions of the arachnoid and pia, respectively, that begin at the junction of the peripheral nerve and dorsal ganglion, within the canal. The intraspinal cyst originally described by Tarlov had a wall that was continuous with the arachnoid and dura of the posterior root/ganglion, whereas the cystic cavity itself occupied the space between the perineurium and endoneurium of the peripheral nerve—hence "perineurial cyst."

Notes

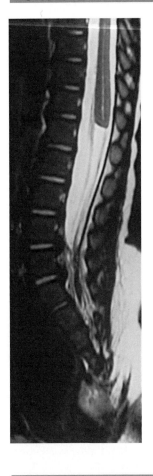

1. Name three anomalies that are part of the syndrome illustrated by the fast-spin-echo T2-weighted image shown here.

2. What metabolic disorder has been linked to this syndrome?

3. Name two of the subcutaneous cystic lesions that have been observed in association with this syndrome.

4. What MR finding has been used to categorize patients with sacral agenesis into two groups with generally different clinical courses?

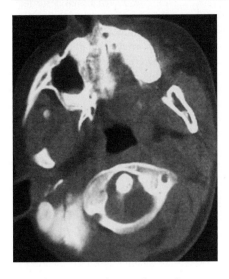 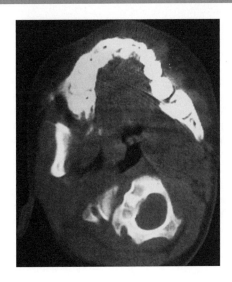

1. What is Grisel's syndrome?

2. What technique is recommended for establishing the diagnosis of atlantoaxial rotatory fixation?

3. List three acquired, nondystonic causes of torticollis.

4. The importance of which structure is emphasized in the Fielding and Hawkins' classification system of rotatory fixation?

Caudal Regression Syndrome

1. Sacral agenesis/dysgenesis, imperforate anus, and bilateral renal aplasia/dysplasia.

2. Maternal diabetes mellitus.

3. Terminal myelocystocele and lipomeningocele.

4. The position of the conus.

References

Barkovich AJ, Raghavan N, Chuang S, Peck WW: The wedge-shaped cord terminus: A radiographic sign of caudal regression. *AJNR Am J Neuroradiol* 10:1223-1231, 1989.

Pang D: Sacral agenesis and caudal spinal cord malformations. *Neurosurgery* 32:755-778, 1993.

Cross-Reference

Neuroradiology: THE REQUISITES, pp 272-276.

Comment

The T2-weighted image shows a blunted, wedge-shaped conus (longer dorsally as a result of a deficiency of anterior horn cells) with a thin central canal extending over at least four vertebral segments. The conus ends approximately at the T12-L1 interspace. A relatively mild sacral dysgenesis is present, with identifiable portions of the sacral vertebra through S4-5. The distal bony canal and thecal sac are narrowed. Patients with sacral agenesis/dysgenesis have been categorized on the basis of conus position: group 1 patients (about 40%) have a high conus terminating cephalic to the inferior end-plate of L1, and group 2 patients (about 60%) have a low conus terminating caudal to L1. In about 90% of group 1 patients the conus has a blunted contour, similar to that shown here. This case is atypical, however, in that group 1 patients tend to have a large sacral defect, with the sacrum ending above S1. In group 2 patients the conus is often elongated as a result of tethering to a thickened filum, lipoma, or myelocystocele. Terminal hydromyelia may be observed in either group. Sacral dysgenesis is relatively mild in group 2 patients; however, their clinical course is more likely to involve neurologic deterioration because of the high percentage of tethered cords. The subcutaneous cystic lesions that have been reported to occur in the setting of sacral agenesis/dysgenesis are terminal myelocystoceles (9% of cases) and lipomeningoceles (6%). Other anomalies reported to be associated with the syndrome of caudal regression include myelomeningocele, diastematomyelia, anterior sacral meningocele, and dermoid.

The syndrome of caudal regression is strongly associated with various maternal diabetic states. About 16% of patients with the syndrome have diabetic mothers, and about 1% of diabetic mothers have offspring with the syndrome. It has been hypothesized that sacral agenesis/dysgenesis may occur as a result of hyperglycemia in a genetically predisposed fetus early in gestation. The insult, like that resulting from various teratogenic agents, may prevent canalization and retrogressive differentiation of the caudal cell mass; alternatively, it may promote excessive retrogression resulting in the sacral deformity and/or anorectal and urogenital malformations. The ventral aspect of the conus may be more affected than the dorsal aspect because the ventrolateral and ventral vascular supply develops earlier, thus allowing enhanced delivery of blood-borne teratogens.

Atlantoaxial Rotatory Deformity

1. Atlantoaxial rotatory deformity resulting from infection (classically nasopharyngeal).

2. CT, with axial images obtained with maximal head rotation to the left and then to the right.

3. Atlantoaxial rotatory dislocation, atlantoaxial anterior subluxation, and C2-3 rotatory dislocation.

4. The transverse ligament.

References

Currier BL: Atlantoaxial rotatory deformities. In: Levine AM, Eismont FJ, Garfin SR, Zigler JE, Eds: *Spine Trauma*. Philadelphia, WB Saunders, 1998, pp 249-267.

Fielding JW, Hawkins RJ: Atlanto-axial rotatory fixation (fixed rotatory subluxation of the atlanto-axial joint). *J Bone Joint Surg Am* 59:37-44, 1977.

Cross-Reference

Neuroradiology: THE REQUISITES, p 500.

Comment

The two CT images represent two sections from the same study, one at the level of C1 (left image) and the other at the level of the C2 body (right image). C1 is rotated clockwise relative to C2 (approximately 45°), and no anterior displacement of C1 on C2 can be seen. Atlantoaxial rotatory deformity refers to a spectrum of disorders. Rotatory deformity may result from infection, trauma, or a variety of other conditions, or it may arise spontaneously (as in this case).

Atlantoaxial rotatory dislocation generally refers to complete dislocation of the C1-2 facet joints. Rotational deformity of the C1-2 joints within the physiologic range of motion has been referred to as an atlantoaxial rotatory displacement by Fielding and Hawkins. In this deformity the joints are not dislocated. If this condition persists and becomes fixed (refractory to nonoperative management), it is then referred to as atlantoaxial rotatory fixation. Recognizing the importance of transverse ligament integrity in determining the degree of canal compromise that can accompany rotational deformities, Fielding and Hawkins described four types of rotatory fixation:

Type I: Rotatory fixation with no anterior displacement (as shown in this case). The transverse ligament is intact, and the odontoid acts as the pivot.

Type II: Rotatory fixation with anterior displacement of 3 to 5 mm. The transverse ligament is mildly deficient or lax, and one facet acts as the pivot.

Type III: Rotatory fixation with anterior displacement of more than 5 mm. The transverse ligament and alar ligaments are deficient.

Type IV: Rotatory fixation with posterior displacement (rare—the only case reported by Fielding and Hawkins was in an adult with rheumatoid arthritis and absence of the dens because of erosion).

Notes

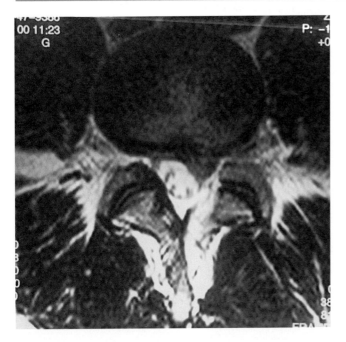 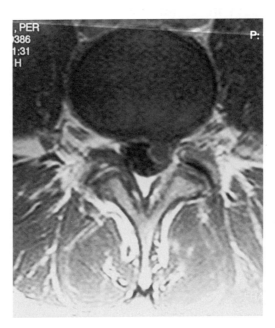

1. List five potential causes of the "failed back surgery" syndrome (FBSS). Which one is most likely responsible for the syndrome in this patient based on the T2- and postcontrast T1-weighted images (L4-5 level) shown here?

2. Are early or delayed (≥30 minutes) postcontrast T1-weighted images better at separating recurrent disk herniation from epidural fibrosis?

3. What percentage of patients undergoing unilateral lumbar laminectomy/diskectomy for disk herniation for the first time are likely to show *intervertebral* disk space enhancement at the surgical level 3 months after surgery (excluding patients with FBSS)?

4. What is the "typical pattern" of postcontrast enhancement in these patients?

Postoperative Recurrent Disk Herniation, Lumbar

1. Epidural fibrosis, recurrent or persistent disk herniation, arachnoiditis, spondylolisthesis, and residual bony stenosis (surgery at the *wrong* level is also a valid answer). Recurrent or persistent disk herniation is most likely in this case.

2. Early.

3. 20%.

4. The typical pattern, as seen on postcontrast T1-weighted *sagittal* images and reported by Ross and colleagues, is "linear horizontal bands of enhancement paralleling the end plates" and converging on the surgical site in the posterior anulus fibrosus.

References

Ross JS: MR imaging of the postoperative lumbar spine. *Magn Reson Imaging Clin N Am* 7:513-524, 1999.
Ross JS, Zepp R, Modic MT: The postoperative lumbar spine: Enhanced MR evaluation of the intervertebral disk. *AJNR Am J Neuroradiol* 17:323-331, 1996.

Cross-Reference

Neuroradiology: THE REQUISITES, pp 470-472.

Comment

The fast-spin-echo T2-weighted image demonstrates asymmetry of the L4 lamina and ligamentum flavum. The ligamentum flavum is disrupted, and part of the left lamina has been removed. The left-sided soft tissue mass contiguous with and isointense to the intervertebral disk could represent a postoperative scar (epidural/peridural fibrosis), recurrent or persistent disk herniation, or a combination of scar plus disk material. On the postcontrast T1-weighted image at the same level, the bulk of the mass does not enhance, compatible with herniation, whereas the thin rim of tissue around the disk does enhance, compatible with mild adjacent scarring. This patient's symptoms were attributed to the recurrent disk herniation.

Typically, a physician who is caring for a patient with symptoms of FBSS wants to know whether the clinical symptoms (recurrent back pain, radiculopathy, and functional incapacitation) are primarily due to "scar or disk." The reported accuracy of postcontrast MR imaging in distinguishing between scar and disk in patients at least 6 weeks after surgery is in the 96% to 100% range. Whether the time elapsed since surgery is months or years, scar consistently enhances on images acquired immediately after injection of contrast material. Because it is avascular, disk does not enhance on these early images. On delayed images (≥30 minutes after injection), disk material may enhance because of diffusion of low-molecular-weight contrast material (gadolinium chelate) into the disk from adjacent scar, especially when the volume of scar is relatively large in comparison with the volume of herniation. A secondary sign that favors scar over recurrent/persistent disk herniation is retraction of the thecal sac toward the region of aberrant epidural soft tissue. The presence of a mass effect is not helpful because both epidural scar and disk herniation can produce this finding.

Notes

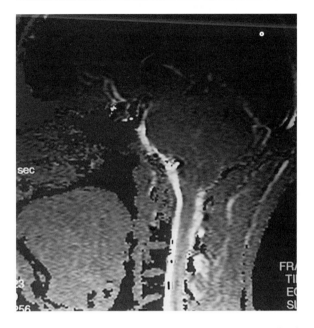 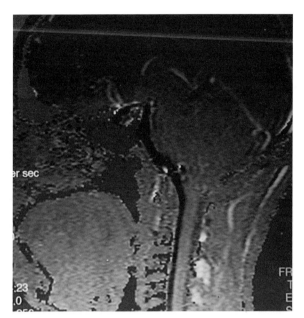

1. What are these images called, and what is the basis for the variation in CSF intensity?

2. What type of pulse sequence is used to obtain such images?

3. What physiologic process is generally thought to be responsible for the signal variation seen here?

4. What is the main use of this technique? Name three lesions that may be better characterized by using this technique.

Acute, Benign Vertebral Fracture

1. Because of the low signal intensity on the diffusion-weighted image (third figure) and secondary findings such as the lack of an associated paraspinal or epidural mass and lack of involvement of the posterior elements.

2. SSFP.

3. When compared with normal vertebral body signal intensity, a pathologic fracture is hyperintense whereas a benign fracture is hypointense or isointense.

4. The "b value." While this is true for images produced with spin-echo and echoplanar sequences, diffusion weighting is determined by a number of factors in addition to "b" for the SSFP sequence.

References

Baur A, Stabler A, Bruning R, et al: Diffusion-weighted MR imaging of bone marrow: Differentiation of benign versus pathologic compression fractures. *Radiology* 207:349–356, 1998.

Buxton RB: Fast diffusion sensitive imaging with steady-state free precession. In: Le Bihan D, Ed: *Diffusion and Perfusion Magnetic Resonance Imaging: Applications to Functional MRI*. New York, Raven, 1995, pp 41–49.

Castillo M, Arbelaez A, Smith JK, Fisher LL: Diffusion-weighted MR imaging offers no advantage over routine noncontrast MR imaging in the detection of vertebral metastases. *AJNR Am J Neuroradiol* 21:948–953, 2000.

Cross-Reference

Neuroradiology: THE REQUISITES, pp 491–493.

Comment

The first two of the three MR images are T1- and T2-weighted spin-echo images. The compressed vertebral body is predominantly hypointense on the T1-weighted image and hypointense or isointense on the T2-weighted image. Very slight retropulsion of the posterior portion of the fragmented vertebral body can be seen. The third image is a diffusion-weighted image obtained with an SSFP pulse sequence and the diffusion gradient (b = 165 sec/mm²) applied only along the read (superior-inferior) axis. For a benign fracture, the diffusion of water protons in the extracellular space is relatively unrestricted. Unrestricted motion in the presence of the diffusion-sensitizing gradient results in loss of signal because of phase dispersion. If motion of the water protons is less restricted than in intact vertebral marrow, the signal intensity of the fractured vertebra will be hypointense, as in this case, in comparison to intact vertebra.

For a pathologic fracture, diffusion of water protons may be relatively restricted because of hypercellularity and tight cell packing in the tumor tissue that has invaded the vertebra. Greater restriction results in less signal loss because phase dispersion is less. Consequently, a pathologically fractured vertebra is hyperintense in comparison with a normal vertebra on the diffusion-weighted image. While this result has been observed for all pathologic fractures reported by some investigators, others have found that pathologic fractures may appear hypointense or hyperintense on diffusion-weighed images obtained with the SSFP sequence. The discrepancy may be due to different tumor cellularity patterns or to differences in implementation of the SSFP technique, and more studies will be needed to determine the efficacy of the technique in distinguishing between benign and pathologic vertebral body fractures.

Notes

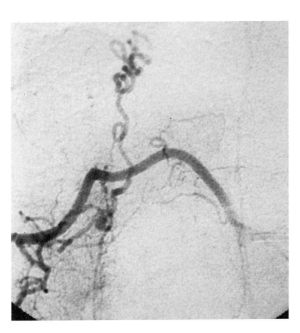
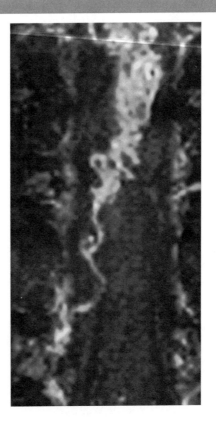

1. What are the four commonly accepted types of spinal arteriovenous malformation (AVM)?
2. Which of these malformations is most common in the general population?
3. Which vessels are shown on both the digital subtraction x-ray angiogram (left) and the postcontrast three-dimensional MR angiogram (right), and why?
4. What are the typical clinical findings and the usual method of treatment for this vascular abnormality?

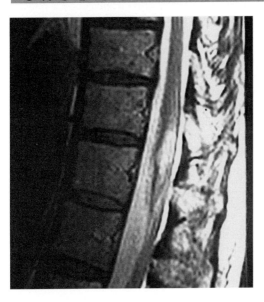
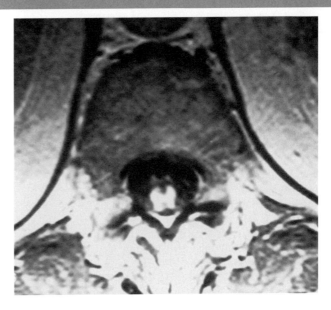

1. Based on the T2-weighted sagittal and the postcontrast T1-weighted axial images, would you consider multiple sclerosis in the differential diagnosis of this conus lesion?
2. Which vessels provide the primary blood supply to the affected region of the cord?
3. How is the diagnosis of arterial infarction usually made?
4. Venous infarction is typically associated with which vascular anomaly?

Dural Arteriovenous Fistula (T11)

1. Type I AVM is a dural arteriovenous (AV) fistula. Type II is an intramedullary glomus-type AVM. Type III is a juvenile-type AVM with intramedullary, extramedullary, and often, extraspinal components. Type IV is an intradural extramedullary AV fistula.

2. Type I AVM.

3. Intradural veins. The tortuous vessel extending from the lower left to the middle of the image is the right T11 medullary (also called radiculomedullary) vein. It is continuous with enlarged veins of the coronal venous plexus on the cord surface. These veins have become enlarged, tortuous, and visible because of shunting of blood through a fistula in the right T11 neural foramen.

4. Dural AV fistula classically occurs in a man between 50 and 70 years old who complains of bilateral leg weakness (spastic paraparesis) and numbness that has been progressive over a period of months to years and more recently has been accompanied by difficulty with urination. The usual treatment is surgical excision of the nidus.

Reference

Bowen BC, Fraser K, Kochan JP, Pattany PM, Green BA, Quencer RM: Spinal dural arteriovenous fistulas: Evaluation with magnetic resonance angiography. *AJNR Am J Neuroradiol* 16:2029-2043, 1995.

Cross-Reference

Neuroradiology: THE REQUISITES, pp 496-498.

Comment

A commonly accepted classification scheme is that of Anson and Spetzler, in which the four types of spinal AVM listed above are described. Type I AVMs are subclassified as types I-A (single feeding artery) and I-B (multiple feeding arteries). The nidus is located within or on the dura of the proximal nerve root sleeve in the neural foramen. These acquired lesions, thought to develop as a result of trauma or venous thrombosis, represent the most common type of spinal AVM. Patients have progressive myelopathy and rarely subarachnoid hemorrhage. Treatment is usually surgical and consists of excision of the dural nidus and interruption of the draining medullary vein. Endovascular therapy with "glue" (NBCA [*N*-butyl cyanoacrylate]) to permanently occlude the fistula is an alternative as long as the anterior spinal artery is not supplied by the segmental artery that is to be occluded.

Type IV AVMs are perimedullary (conus/cauda equina) fistulas. They may vary in severity from type IV-A (slow flow, single feeding artery, moderately enlarged spinal veins), which is treated surgically, to type IV-C (high flow, multiple feeders, markedly dilated veins), which is treated endovascularly with coils, particles, and/or balloons. Patients, who generally range in age from 2 to 40 years, may have progressive myelopathy, subarachnoid hemorrhage (up to 50% of cases), or acute paraplegia without hemorrhage. Type II and type III AVMs are discussed in association with other cases in this book.

Notes

Conus Medullaris Infarction

1. No, the lesion involves primarily central gray matter, not peripheral white matter.

2. The sulcal (or sulcocommissural) branches of the anterior spinal artery.

3. On clinical grounds. Arterial occlusion is often difficult to verify by spinal angiography.

4. Dural arteriovenous fistula.

Reference

Yawad ME, Rivera V, Crawford S: Spinal cord ischemia after resection of thoracoabdominal aortic aneurysms: MR findings in 24 patients. *AJNR Am J Neuroradiol* 11:987-991, 1990.

Cross-Reference

Neuroradiology: THE REQUISITES, pp 495-496.

Comment

Blood is supplied to the cord by the sulcal branches of the anterior spinal artery, which itself is primarily supplied by the artery of Adamkiewicz in the conus region, and by radial perforating branches of the pial arterial plexus on the cord surface. The anterior spinal artery supplies approximately the anterior two thirds of the cord and most of the central gray matter. Hypoperfusion in this vascular distribution, as may occur from pathologic changes in the descending aorta (aneurysm, thrombosis, dissection) or from small vessel vasculitides, can result in conus infarction. Spin-echo MR findings are cord enlargement and hyperintense signal on T2-weighted images initially (8 hours to several days), with or without gadolinium enhancement, followed by cord atrophy later (months). Abnormal signal and enhancement may demonstrate a double-dot ("owl's eyes") pattern in the region of the anterior horns, an H-shaped pattern involving the central gray matter, or a more diffuse pattern involving both gray and white matter. Viral infections or neurodegenerative diseases affecting the central gray matter can mimic one of these patterns on T2-weighted imaging. The diffuse pattern of signal abnormality and enhancement may be difficult to distinguish from venous infarction, which results from venous congestion associated with a dural arteriovenous fistula or thrombophlebitis.

Notes

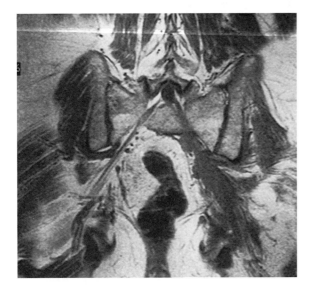
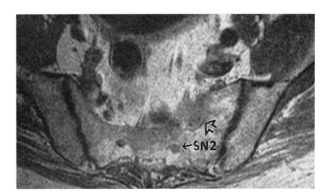

1. What extrapelvic imaging findings on the precontrast coronal and postcontrast axial T1-weighted images are consistent with S1 and S2 lesions in this patient with sciatica?

2. List three extraspinal causes of sciatica.

3. How might a *lumbar* neural foraminal lesion be distinguished from a lumbosacral plexus lesion on the basis of muscle atrophy and fatty replacement detected on T1-weighted images?

4. Which normal structures in the anterior sacral foramina show gadolinium enhancement on MR images?

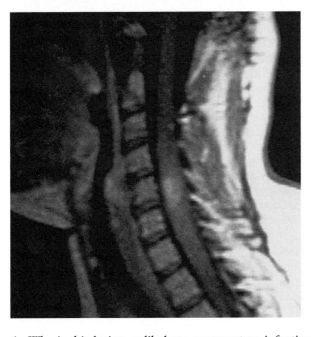
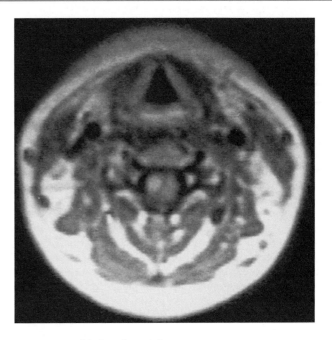

1. Why is this lesion unlikely to represent an infectious process or multiple sclerosis?

2. Hemorrhagic lesions occur in which demyelinating disease?

3. What is the incidence of leptomeningeal and intramedullary metastatic disease?

4. Are CSF cytology studies likely to be positive or negative?

Metastatic Tumor Infiltration of Sacral Nerves and Plexus*

1. Atrophy and fatty replacement involving the left gluteus maximus, which is innervated by the anterior rami of the L5 through S2 roots via the inferior gluteal nerve.

2. Paraspinal lesion (e.g., lymphoma), sacral plexus lesion (e.g., metastasis, direct invasion by endometrial or colorectal carcinoma, endometriosis), and sciatic nerve lesion or compression (e.g., nerve sheath tumor, femoral fracture or dislocation, hematoma).

3. The lumbar nerve lesion affects both the lower extremity muscles (anterior ramus denervation) and the paraspinal muscles (posterior ramus denervation), whereas only the lower extremity muscles are affected by a plexus lesion.

4. Veins.

Reference

Bowen BC: Lumbosacral plexus. In: Stark DD, Bradley WG Jr, Eds: *Magnetic Resonance Imaging*, third edition, Vol 3. Philadelphia, Mosby-Year Book, 1998, pp 1907-1916.

Cross-Reference

Neuroradiology: THE REQUISITES, p 491.

Comment

Sciatica is a term used to describe a syndrome of acute pain radiating into the leg. The sciatica is usually in the distribution of S1 (down the back of the leg to the heel) and/or L5 (down the lateral surface of the leg to the instep) because these two roots are the ones most commonly affected by degenerative disk disease. The symptoms, however, may be mimicked by lesions in the pelvis involving the sacral plexus or lesions in the gluteal/upper thigh region involving the sciatic nerve. In this case, the coronal T1-weighted image demonstrates the course of the normal right S1 root exiting the anterior foramen and then continuing inferiorly and laterally to join the sacral plexus (at the parasagittal level of the sacroiliac joint) and continuing into the upper portion of the thigh as the sciatic nerve. The corresponding left neural structures, however, are infiltrated by a mass that tracks along the left S1 root superiorly. The postcontrast axial image shows enhancement of the mass enveloping the S1 root and eroding the anterior surface of the sacrum *(open arrow)*. The left S2 root (SN2) in the neural foramen is also enhanced and enlarged in comparison with the normal right side. This finding is consistent with retrograde, perineural spread of tumor, which was proved by biopsy to be metastatic from a primary lung carcinoma.

---

*Figures for Case 59 from Bowen BC: Lumbosacral plexus. In: Stark DD, Bradley WG Jr, Eds: *Magnetic Resonance Imaging*, third edition, Vol 3. Philadelphia, Mosby-Year Book, 1998, pp 1907-1916.

Notes

Intramedullary Metastasis (Melanoma)

1. Both figures are precontrast T1-weighted images. The lesion is hyperintense and thus has a shortened T1, which may result from the presence of fat or paramagnetic substances such as methemoglobin (hemorrhage) or melanin (metastatic melanoma). These properties, plus cord enlargement, suggest a tumor or vascular lesion rather than multiple sclerosis or an inflammatory/infectious process.

2. Acute disseminated encephalomyelitis.

3. Approximately 3% of patients with metastatic disease have leptomeningeal and/or intramedullary metastases.

4. Negative.

References

Markus JB: Magnetic resonance imaging of intramedullary spinal cord metastases. *Clin Imaging* 20:238-242, 1996.

Premkumar A, Marincola F, Taubenberger J, et al: Metastatic melanoma: Corrrelation of MRI characteristics and histopathology. *J Magn Reson Imaging* 6:190-194, 1996.

Cross-Reference

Neuroradiology: THE REQUISITES, pp 81, 487-489.

Comment

Melanoma metastases may have different combinations of signal intensity on T1- and T2-weighted images: (1) high/variable (but often low) for melanotic lesions, (2) low/high for amelanotic lesions, (3) high/high for subacute hemorrhagic lesions, and (4) low(iso)/low for acute hemorrhagic lesions. Several investigators have found a strong correlation between melanin content and T1 shortening. In the example shown here, the peripheral intramedullary mass had high signal intensity on T1-weighted images and low signal intensity on T2-weighted images (not shown), consistent with melanotic metastasis. Intramedullary metastases are uncommon (on the order of 1% of tumor patients) and result from either hematogenous or CSF spread. Leptomeningeal tumor may extend into the cord via Virchow-Robin spaces and be manifested as intramedullary masses. Neoplasms that tend to metastasize to the spinal cord or leptomeninges from outside the CNS are lung and breast carcinoma and melanoma. Lymphoma and leukemia may also involve the cord.

Notes

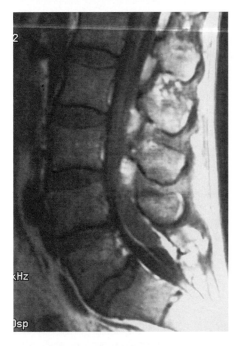
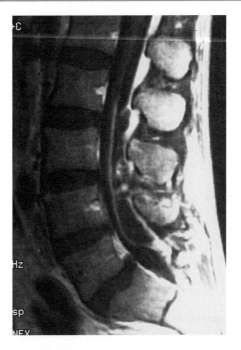

1. In which space is this lesion most likely located?

2. What patterns of enhancement can be observed with this type of lesion?

3. Besides the mass effect, what other mechanism has been proposed to account for the symptomatology and lesion appearance?

4. How does this lesion differ from metastatic tumor?

C A S E   6 2

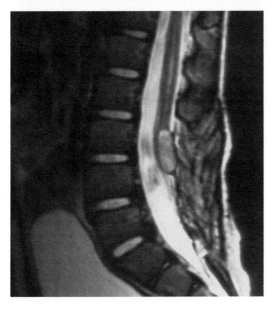
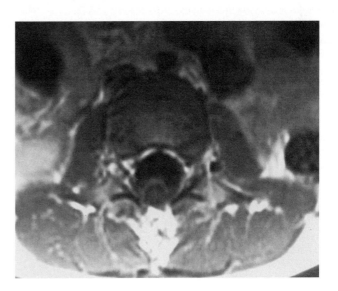

1. Based on the T2-weighted sagittal and postcontrast T1-weighted axial images shown above, is this lesion congenital or acquired?

2. If congenital, is it more likely to be a teratoma, dermoid, or epidermoid?

3. What congenital midline soft tissue defect is most likely to occur in association with this mass?

4. Is this lesion intramedullary or extramedullary?

C A S E 6 1

Epidural Abscess, Lumbar

1. Dorsal epidural space.

2. Three patterns of enhancement have been described: homogeneous, peripheral, and a combination of these two.

3. Thrombophlebitis of the epidural veins.

4. Epidural metastatic tumor is more localized and associated with focal bone invasion and destruction.

Reference

Post MJD, Bowen BC, Sze G: Magnetic resonance imaging of spinal infection. *Rheum Dis Clin North Am* 17:773–794, 1991.

Cross-Reference

Neuroradiology: THE REQUISITES, p 479.

Comment

Epidural abscess may occur from hematogenous dissemination, secondary infection of an epidural hematoma, or extension of vertebral osteomyelitis/diskitis. Identification of the epidural location of the lesion is based on irregular disruption (L4 through S1 in the precontrast T1-weighted image) of the normal segmental distribution of high–signal intensity epidural fat (L1 and L2). Potentially, an intradural lesion could compress epidural fat and mimic an epidural lesion. The peripheral pattern of enhancement in this case is consistent with a mature abscess; however, the infection is often imaged during the cellulitis stage of the disease and demonstrates relatively homogeneous enhancement rather than cavity formation. Epidural abscess may have a significant hemorrhagic component, either because of a preexisting hematoma or because of hypothesized rupture of epidural veins as the infectious mass expands. Involvement of epidural veins by the inflammatory process can potentially lead to septic thrombophlebitis, which by extension to the spinal cord veins can result in cord edema and infarction. Direct compression on neural tissue, however, is considered to be the major cause of symptoms.

Notes

C A S E 6 2

Epidermoid Cyst

1. The low position and tethering of the conus, with syrinx, suggest a congenital lesion.

2. Epidermoid, because this lesion does not have a short T1 component as seen with teratoma and some dermoids.

3. Dorsal dermal sinus.

4. Probably both, as has been reported for most epidermoids and dermoids associated with a dermal sinus.

Reference

Naidich TP, Zimmerman RA, McLone DG, Raybaud CA, Altman NR, Braffman BH: Congenital anomalies of the spine and spinal cord. In: Atlas SW, Ed: *Magnetic Resonance Imaging of the Brain and Spine.* Philadelphia, Lippincott-Raven, 1996, pp 1265–1337.

Cross-Reference

Neuroradiology: THE REQUISITES, p 484.

Comment

The signal characteristics of epidermoid and dermoid cysts are variable and depend on their keratin, collagen, cholesterol, and water composition. This variability probably explains why the cyst is not isointense relative to CSF on the T1- or T2-weighted images. Minimal or no contrast enhancement in the wall of the cyst, as shown here, is typical. It is difficult to determine whether the cyst is intramedullary or extramedullary, and sometimes these lesions have both components. Fifteen percent of all CNS epidermoid and dermoid tumors are located in the spine. Spinal epidermoid and dermoid tumors occur with approximately equal frequency. The majority of epidermoids are found in the lumbar region, whereas the majority of dermoids are in the thoracolumbar region. Twenty to 25% of cases (depending on various reports) have an associated dermal sinus. Epidermoid cysts may be acquired rather than congenital and result from implantation of viable skin elements during back surgery or spinal puncture.

Notes

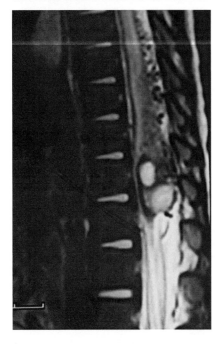 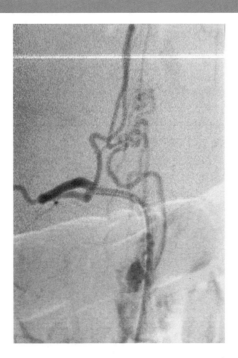

1. Is this patient likely to be older or younger than 50 years?
2. Does this lesion have a preferred location along the spinal axis?
3. How does the venous drainage of this lesion differ from that of a dural arteriovenous (AV) fistula?
4. List at least three findings on selective spinal angiography that can affect the management of spinal vascular malformations.

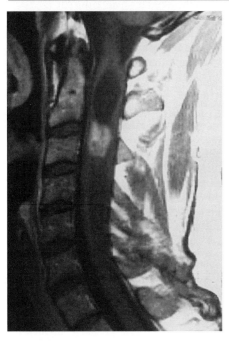 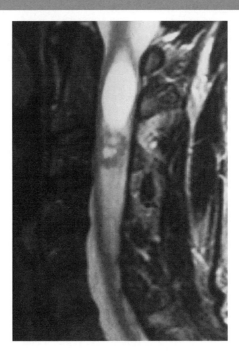

1. What is the cause of the cord enlargement at C2 on the T2-weighted and postcontrast T1-weighted images?
2. Do spinal ependymomas occur earlier or later in life than intracranial ependymomas?
3. Is vigorous enhancement more likely with ependymoma or astrocytoma?
4. Approximately what percentage of ependymomas demonstrate associated cysts?

Intramedullary Arteriovenous Malformation (Glomus Type at T12)

1. Younger.

2. No, as opposed to spinal dural AV fistulas, which are usually located between the T4 and L3 vertebral levels.

3. The direction of blood flow in the medullary (or radiculomedullary) vein is reversed with a dural fistula in comparison to a glomus AV malformation (AVM).

4. Management, in terms of surgery and/or embolization, can be affected by any of the following findings: the feeding artery originates from the anterior spinal artery, the AVM envelops the anterior spinal artery, a perinidal aneurysm is present, or a metameric angiomatosis (Cobb's syndrome with angiomas of the skin, vertebra, and spinal cord) is present.

Reference

Bao Y-H, Ling F: Classification and therapeutic modalities of spinal vascular malformations in 80 patients. *Neurosurgery* 40:75-81, 1997.

Cross-Reference

Neuroradiology: THE REQUISITES, pp 496-498.

Comment

A glomus AVM of the spinal cord (type II AVM, Anson-Spetzler classification) is supplied by branches of the anterior and/or posterior spinal arteries. The intramedullary nidus drains into the coronal venous plexus on the cord surface, which in turn drains through a medullary vein or veins to the extradural space in an antegrade manner. In comparison, the flow from the nidus of a dural AV fistula is retrograde through the medullary vein and subsequently passes into the veins on the cord surface. Patients with a glomus AVM are usually younger than 50 years and have an abrupt onset of myelopathy. Fifty percent of patients have evidence of subarachnoid hemorrhage. In those amenable to treatment, the goal is complete surgical excision of the nidus, yet complete excision may require preoperative embolization of surgically inaccessible arteries or occlusion of a feeding artery aneurysm. In juvenile (type III) AVM the nidus is more diffuse, the prognosis is worse, and treatment consists of combined surgical and endovascular therapy, the goal of which is to achieve partial resection or reduction of AVM volume. These lesions occur in children and young adults.

Notes

Ependymoma With Associated Cysts, Cervical

1. Rostral cyst.

2. Later.

3. Ependymomas are highly vascular and thus enhance markedly.

4. Approximately 30% to 50%, depending on the definition of "cyst."

Reference

Kahan H, Sklar EM, Post MJ, Bruce JH: MR characteristics of histopathologic subtypes of spinal ependymoma. *AJNR Am J Neuroradiol* 17:143-150, 1996.

Cross-Reference

Neuroradiology: THE REQUISITES, pp 486-487.

Comment

In patients with spinal cord ependymoma, three types of "cyst" have been described:

1. Intratumoral cysts, which are lined by abnormal glia, contain blood or xanthochromic fluid, and have enhancing margins on postcontrast T1-weighted images.

2. Rostral or caudal cysts, sometimes called "tumor cysts," are cord cavitations at the margins of the tumor. These cysts are typically glial lined, are filled with CSF-like fluid, and do not enhance on postcontrast T1-weighted images (as in this case).

3. Reactive dilatation of the central canal. This type is recognized by its central location within the cord and its location beyond the tumor margins. Distinction between rostral/caudal cysts and reactive dilatation of the central canal may be difficult, and some authors do not make a clear distinction between these cysts.

Based on autopsy studies, 46% of ependymomas have associated cystic cavities of the spinal cord. It is important to differentiate intratumoral cysts from the other two types of cyst on imaging because intratumoral cysts should be excised with the tumor whereas rostral/caudal cysts do not need to be excised. They contain no tumor cells and may be aspirated and drained. When compared with intratumoral cysts, rostral/caudal cysts and central canal dilatation are more likely to show evidence of intracystic CSF motion (i.e., signal loss) on MR images acquired without motion compensation.

Notes

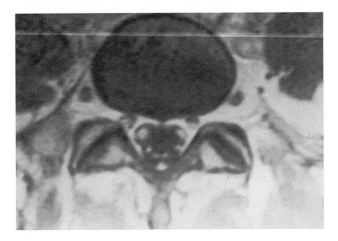

1. In what percentage of unoperated patients are you likely to detect idiopathic nerve root enhancement on postcontrast (0.1 mmol/kg gadolinium chelate) T1-weighted images—less than or greater than 10%?

2. Which primary CNS neoplasms tend to spread via the subarachnoid space?

3. What finding on this postcontrast T1-weighted axial image (L4-5 level) favors leptomeningeal tumor over infectious arachnoiditis?

4. Which portions of spinal nerve roots show enhancement in all individuals?

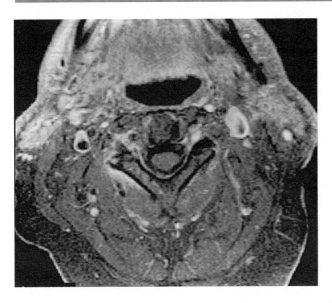 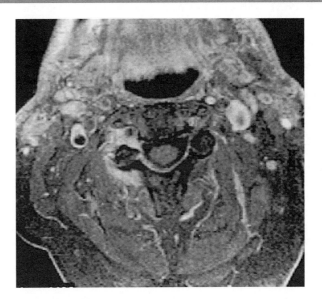

1. What are the most common causes of a paraspinous/epidural mass?

2. List three primary soft tissue tumors that are in the differential diagnosis of a paraspinous mass.

3. Do the signal abnormalities on the postcontrast, fat saturation T1-weighted images involve only the paraspinous/epidural region?

4. Would you perform a biopsy on this lesion?

Drop Metastases (Glioblastoma Multiforme)

1. Less than 10%.

2. Glioblastoma multiforme, ependymoma, primitive neuroectodermal tumor, and germ cell tumor.

3. Striking enhancement of several individual nerve roots without gross clumping of roots favors leptomeningeal tumor. Sarcoid can mimic the appearance of tumor.

4. Dorsal root ganglia.

Reference

Gomori JM, Heching N, Siegal T: Leptomeningeal metastases: Evaluation by gadolinium enhanced spinal magnetic resonance imaging. *J Neurooncol* 36:55-60, 1998.

Cross-Reference

Neuroradiology: THE REQUISITES, pp 487-488.

Comment

Postcontrast individual nerve root enhancement on T1-weighted images may be seen in unoperated individuals and occurs as a result of disruption of the blood-nerve barrier for any of a number of reasons: compression (disk herniation), ischemia, demyelination, and axonal degeneration. In some cases, linear radicular enhancement may be due to filling of a great medullary (radiculomedullary) vein paralleling the course of the corresponding nerve root and may mimic true root enhancement. Enhancement of multiple, clumped roots of the cauda equina is characteristic of lumbar arachnoiditis, which can result from infection, trauma, surgery, or myelography. On precontrast scans, T2-weighted images are more sensitive than T1-weighted images in detecting clumped nerve roots because adhesions of only a few nerves can be detected by enlargement and displacement of the normally symmetric low-signal dots within the high-signal CSF. Postcontrast T1-weighted MR imaging, without or with fat suppression, is the examination of choice for the detection of leptomeningeal metastases. In one study, leptomeningeal metastases were detected on postcontrast images in approximately 50% of high-risk patients with negative initial CSF cytology or no spinal symptoms. Of the adult gliomas, the one that most commonly spreads via the CSF is glioblastoma multiforme. Subarachnoid seeding occurs when tumor breaks through the ependyma into the ventricular system.

Notes

Degenerative Facet Disease, Cervical

1. Metastases (breast, lung, prostate, kidney), lymphoma, and less often, leukemia, neural crest tumors (neuroblastoma, ganglioneuroblastoma, ganglioneuroma), and inflammatory/infectious disease (granulomatous disease).

2. Malignant fibrous histiocytoma, liposarcoma, and desmoid fibromatosis.

3. No. Abnormal enhancement of the right C2 lamina can be seen.

4. Depends on the clinical picture, previous studies, and alternative imaging such as CT or bone scan. CT was performed after MR imaging, and the findings were consistent with degenerative disease of the right C2-3 facet joint. A study 1 month later showed no new findings; however, the patient, a surgeon, became concerned and insisted on a biopsy.

Reference

Fletcher G, Haughton VM, Ho KC, Yu SW: Age-related changes in the cervical facet joints: Studies with cryomicrotomy, MR, and CT. *AJR Am J Roentgenol* 154:817-820, 1990.

Cross-Reference

Neuroradiology: THE REQUISITES, pp 460-470.

Comment

Degeneration of the facet joint, which has a thin synovial lining, is characterized by loss of cartilage from the articular surface. Subsequent degenerative changes include subarticular erosions, sclerosis of bone, and hypertrophy. Anteriorly, the facet joint has no capsule and no border except the ligamentum flavum. Posteriorly, the joint has a thick fibrous capsule. This capsule covers the joint space and portions of the adjacent articular processes. Osseous and cartilaginous changes in the degenerated joint are well shown by CT, but the chronic inflammation induced in the capsule and adjacent soft tissues is better demonstrated by MR imaging, especially when fat saturation techniques are used.

Notes

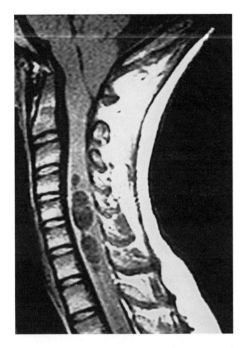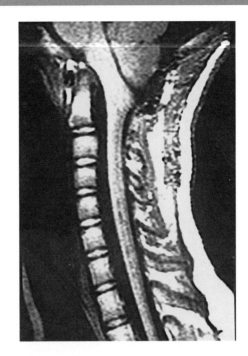

1. Name three associated congenital osseous abnormalities.
2. What is the incidence of associated syringohydromyelia?
3. What measurement of tonsillar ectopia correlates with a significant increase in clinical symptoms?
4. What is the treatment of choice?

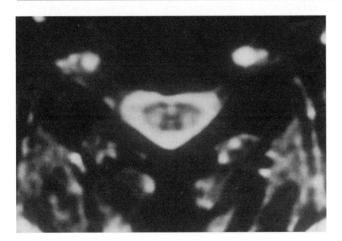

1. Is this patient more likely to have pain or weakness?
2. Atrophy of which portion of the cord may be evident?
3. Would you recommend MR imaging of the brain? Why or why not?
4. On physical examination, is this patient likely to have pure upper motor neuron, pure lower motor neuron, or combined upper and lower motor neuron signs?

C A S E 6 7

Chiari I Malformation, Pretreatment and Posttreatment

1. Klippel-Feil anomalies, occipitalization of the atlas, and omovertebral bones.

2. 20% to 73% (the lower percentage is more likely correct).

3. When the tips of the tonsils extend more than 5 mm below a line drawn from the basion to the opisthion.

4. Suboccipital craniectomy and duraplasty to achieve tonsillar decompression.

References

Barkovich AJ, Wippold FJ, Sherman JL, Citrin CM: Significance of cerebellar tonsillar ectopia on MR. *AJNR Am J Neuroradiol* 7:795-799, 1986.

Bindal AK, Dunsker SB, Tew JM Jr: Chiari I malformation: Classification and management. *Neurosurgery* 37:1069-1074, 1995.

Cross-Reference

Neuroradiology: THE REQUISITES, pp 261-262.

Comment

The Chiari I malformation is associated with inferior displacement of the cerebellar tonsils and sometimes the inferior vermis, with a normal location of the fourth ventricle and brainstem. Tonsillar ectopia less than 5 mm is of uncertain significance. The incidence of clinical symptoms increases markedly with ectopia greater than 5 mm. The most common cause of Chiari I malformation is dysgenesis at the craniocervical junction. Other causes of tonsillar ectopia include intrauterine or postnatal hydrocephalus and secondary or acquired forms of basilar invagination (referred to as basilar impression). Chiari I–associated syringohydromyelia is usually cervical in location, whereas a Chiari II–associated syrinx is more often seen in the lower thoracic or conus region of a tethered cord. Syringohydromyelia associated with Chiari I usually first occurs later in life and has been attributed to abnormal CSF flow at the foramen magnum. Current treatment is based on the presence of signs and symptoms of brainstem compression, syringohydromyelia, or both. Resection of the posterior margin of the foramen magnum from condyle to condyle, cervical laminectomy to expose the caudal limit of tonsillar herniation, and duraplasty produce striking improvement in symptoms resulting from brainstem compression. The procedure also leads to stabilization or improvement in symptoms attributable to syringohydromyelia, as in this case, in which posterior brainstem decompression resulted in nearly complete resolution of the syrinx.

Notes

C A S E 6 8

Amyotrophic Lateral Sclerosis

1. Weakness, because the signal abnormality primarily involves the lateral columns and the bilaterality suggests amyotrophic lateral sclerosis (ALS).

2. Anterior horn cell region.

3. Yes, to look for bilateral abnormal hyperintensity in the corticospinal tracts on long recovery time (TR) dual-echo images, which would support a diagnosis of ALS.

4. Combined upper and lower motor neuron signs.

References

Mascalchi M, Salvi F, Valzania F, Marcacci G, Bartolozzi C, Tassinari CA: Corticospinal tract degeneration in motor neuron disease. *AJNR Am J Neuroradiol* 16:878-880, 1995.

Waragai M, Shinotoh H, Hayashi M, Hattori T: High signal intensity on T1-weighted MRI of the anterolateral column of the spinal cord in amyotrophic lateral sclerosis. *J Neurol Neurosurg Psychiatry* 62:88-91, 1997.

Cross-Reference

Neuroradiology: THE REQUISITES, p 236.

Comment

ALS is a syndrome of upper and lower motor neuron dysfunction of the arms, legs, and bulbar and/or respiratory motor systems that slowly progresses over months to years in adults without involvement of any other part of the nervous system or the presence of any specific cause. Histopathologic examination shows selective degeneration of the somatic motor neurons of the brainstem nuclei and spinal cord (anterior horn cells), as well as the large pyramidal neurons of the motor cortex. Associated degeneration of the corticospinal tracts has been tracked in postmortem specimens from the cerebral cortex to the conus medullaris. Correspondingly, high signal intensity of the corticospinal tracts on T2-weighted images has been tracked from the centrum semiovale to the lower cervical spine in patients with ALS. The symmetry of the hyperintensity distinguishes these findings from multiple sclerosis and other demyelinating diseases, as well as wallerian degeneration resulting from infarction. High signal intensity on T1-weighted images in the anterolateral columns of the spinal cord has also been reported.

Notes

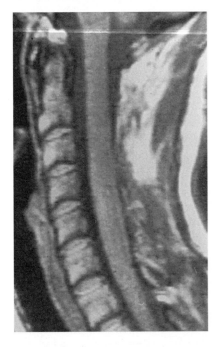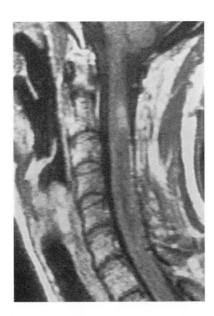

1. Based on the precontrast and postcontrast images in this patient with rapidly progressive cervical myelopathy and normal CSF analysis, would you recommend biopsy as soon as possible?

2. What is transverse myelitis?

3. Name three diseases that cause this condition.

4. In what disease or syndrome are transverse myelitis and optic neuritis associated?

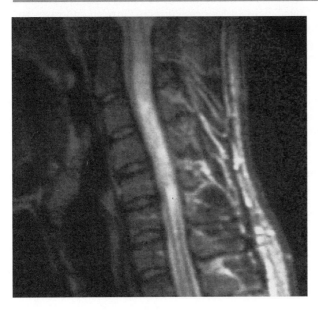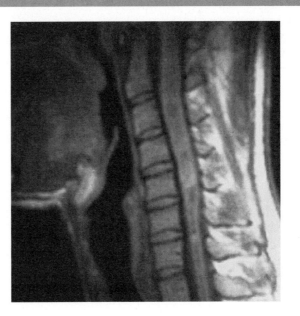

1. List five causes of spinal cord enlargement.

2. What is the most common spinal cord tumor in patients between 20 and 50 years of age?

3. True or false: Ependymomas and astrocytomas have a similar distribution in terms of frequency of occurrence along the spinal axis.

4. Which of these two types of tumor is more likely to appear infiltrating and unresectable?

Acute Multiple Sclerosis

1. No, the diagnosis of acute multiple sclerosis should be considered and MR imaging of the brain recommended initially.

2. Transverse myelitis is a clinical diagnosis. It is characterized by the acute or subacute development of paraplegia, occasionally asymmetric, associated with back or neck pain and sensory loss.

3. Multiple sclerosis, acute disseminated encephalomyelitis, and lupus erythematosus.

4. Devic's disease.

References

Campi A, Filippi M, Comi G, et al: Acute transverse myelopathy: Spinal and cranial MR study with clinical follow-up. *AJNR Am J Neuroradiol* 16:115-123, 1995.

Hittmair K, Mallek R, Prayer D, Schindler EG, Kollegger H: Spinal cord lesions in patients with multiple sclerosis: Comparison of MR pulse sequences. *AJNR Am J Neuroradiol* 17:1555-1565, 1996.

Cross-Reference

Neuroradiology: THE REQUISITES, pp 206, 480-481.

Comment

The findings of cord enlargement and mild hypointensity over several levels on the precontrast T1-weighted image and focal enhancement on the postcontrast image reflect the presence of edema and breakdown of the blood-cord barrier. The observations are nonspecific and may result from a neoplasm, such as astrocytoma, or from various inflammatory conditions, such as those causing transverse myelitis. Indeed, in this case a laminectomy and cord biopsy were performed because of suspicion of tumor, and the diagnosis was demyelinating disease. An important finding in the midsagittal, postcontrast image is that enhancement is posteriorly located, that is, in the region of the posterior columns. This pattern should raise suspicion of multiple sclerosis, in which demyelinating lesions preferentially occur in the posterior and lateral segments of the cord. Because only 15% to 20% of patients with multiple sclerosis have isolated spinal cord involvement, MR imaging of the brain is likely to show evidence of demyelinating lesions, thus avoiding the need for cord biopsy to rule out neoplasm.

Multiple sclerosis is one of several diseases or disorders that can cause the constellation of clinical findings referred to as transverse myelitis. Often, transverse myelitis is due to an allergic reaction related to previous infection or vaccination or to direct infection by a virus. The midthoracic cord is commonly involved.

Notes

Astrocytoma

1. Primary spinal cord tumor, multiple sclerosis, sarcoid, syringomyelia, and acute infarction.

2. Ependymoma.

3. False. Approximately 75% of astrocytomas occur in the cervicothoracic cord, whereas about 60% of ependymomas occur in the conus medullaris and cauda equina/filum terminale region.

4. Astrocytoma.

Reference

Epstein FJ, Farmer J-P, Freed D: Adult intramedullary astrocytomas of the spinal cord. *J Neurosurg* 77:335-339, 1992.

Cross-Reference

Neuroradiology: THE REQUISITES, pp 485-486.

Comment

Typically, patients with spinal cord astrocytoma are initially evaluated in the third to fifth decades of life for neck, back, or leg pain; lower (and/or upper) extremity weakness; and spasticity. Approximately 75% of these lesions are found in the cervical or thoracic spine, 20% in the conus region, and 5% in the filum terminale. Spinal cord astrocytomas are usually less malignant than brain astrocytomas, with approximately 50% being grade 1 and less than 10% being grade 4. On histopathologic and MR examination, they have an infiltrating appearance and are more likely than ependymomas to involve the full diameter of the cord. On MR imaging, cord astrocytomas involve multiple levels, have a heterogeneous signal, and are hypointense relative to cord on T1-weighted images and hyperintense on T2-weighted images. In addition to tumoral replacement of cord tissue, heterogeneous signal results from the presence of edema, intratumoral cyst, hemorrhage, and/or syringomyelia. These tumors generally show inhomogeneous gadolinium enhancement that is not limited to gray or white matter, in distinction to acute multiple sclerosis, which often shows primarily enhancement of white matter tracts. Enhancement localizes the main portion of the tumor but does not necessarily define its microscopic boundaries. On serial postsurgical MR images, progressive cord enlargement and increasing cord enhancement are regarded as signs of tumor recurrence.

Notes

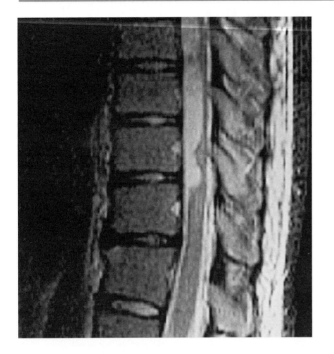 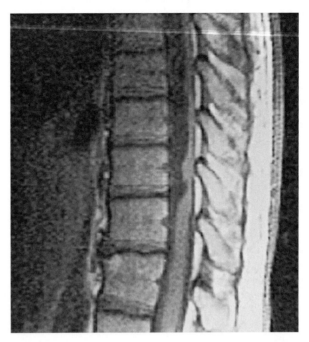

1. Would you describe the cord as atrophic or compressed?

2. Are the patient's symptoms likely to be due to a congenital or an acquired process?

3. If acquired, list four etiologies.

4. What additional imaging studies would be diagnostically useful?

Arachnoid Cyst (Postinfectious), Thoracic

1. Compressed.

2. Acquired, because congenital arachnoid cysts are predominantly posterior in location and no scalloping of bone or other evidence of a long-standing congenital process is present.

3. Chronic infectious meningitis, previous trauma, spine surgery, or myelography with iophendylate (Pantopaque).

4. Cine-MR flow study and/or myelography with postmyelographic CT (early and delayed scans).

References

Shimizu H, Tominaga T, Takahashi A, Yoshimoto T: Cine MR imaging of spinal intradural arachnoid cysts. *Neurosurgery* 41:95–100, 1997.

Sklar E, Quencer RM, Green BA, Montalvo BM, Post MJ: Acquired spinal subarachnoid cysts: Evaluation with MR, CT myelography, and intraoperative sonography. *AJNR Am J Neuroradiol* 10:1097–1104, 1989.

Cross-Reference

Neuroradiology: THE REQUISITES, p 484.

Comment

In a patient with apparent enlargement of the subarachnoid space and decreased cord size, one must distinguish between cord atrophy and cord compression by a cyst. Atrophy is more likely when flow artifacts (caused by normal CSF motion) are observed in the subarachnoid space. Cord compression is more likely when these artifacts are absent and when the cord exhibits a flattened, scalloped, or lobulated contour (as in this case), right-left displacement, or tenting. Also, posterior displacement of the cord in a region of kyphosis or anterior displacement in a region of lordosis suggests that a mass is present. Cord or nerve root compression may be due to an acquired subarachnoid cyst or a congenital arachnoid cyst (both sometimes referred to as an "arachnoid" cyst) or to an infectious cyst with CSF-equivalent signal intensity. Patients who have a history of trauma, myelography with Pantopaque, spine surgery, chronic infectious meningitis, or other inflammatory diseases such as ankylosing spondylitis are at increased risk for arachnoiditis, adhesions, and altered CSF flow dynamics. These conditions probably predispose to the formation of a subarachnoid cyst or cysts, as well as a syrinx, although the pathogenesis remains to be proved. Congenital arachnoid cysts may be located deep (intradural) or superficial to the dura (extradural) or be positioned within the dura. Intradural cysts (type III spinal meningeal cyst) probably arise by loculation of arachnoid trabeculae, particularly in and adjacent to the septum posticum in the thoracic region (80%). CNS cysticercosis and hydatid disease can produce infectious cysts that have CSF-equivalent signal on MR imaging.

Normal CSF pulsations in the subarachnoid space cause localized areas of decreased signal on spin-echo T2-weighted images, and they cause decreased or increased signal on gradient-echo T2*-weighted images without or with motion compensation, respectively. The gradient-echo images can be ac- quired as part of a cardiac-gated protocol and then displayed in a closed-loop cine mode to demonstrate CSF (and cord) motion. This motion may be absent or asynchronous in regions where the subarachnoid space is obliterated by the presence of a cyst. Sometimes, myelography and postmyelographic CT are better than MR imaging at demonstrating the presence of subarachnoid cysts. Filling defects present on the initial images may show early or delayed opacification, depending on the rate of entry of contrast into the cyst or cysts.

Notes

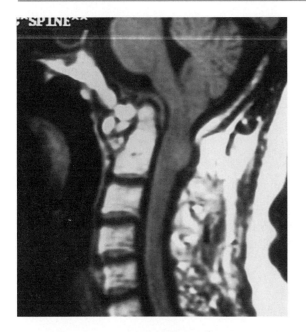

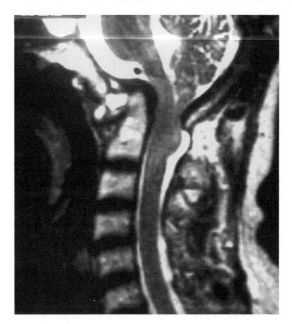

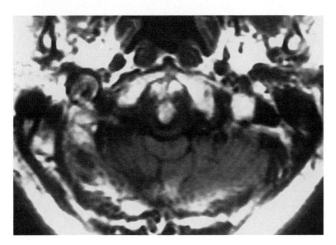

1. Which term best describes the imaging findings: platybasia, basilar impression, or basilar invagination?

2. From these images, which craniometric measurement is clearly abnormal: Welcker's basal angle, the Wackenheim clivus baseline, or the atlantooccipital joint axis angle?

3. Which of the following are not associated with basilar invagination: occiput, atlas, or axis anomalies?

4. Chamberlain's line is drawn between which two anatomic landmarks? What is the significance of this line?

Basilar Invagination

1. Basilar invagination.

2. Wackenheim clivus baseline.

3. Axis anomalies.

4. Between the posterior edge of the hard palate and the opisthion. Usually, the tip of the odontoid process and the anterior arch of the atlas lie below this line.

Reference

Smoker WRK: Craniovertebral junction: Normal anatomy, craniometry, and congenital anomalies. *Radiographics* 14:255–277, 1994.

Cross-Reference

Neuroradiology: THE REQUISITES, p 264.

Comment

Basilar invagination is a primary developmental anomaly that usually results from an underlying abnormality of the occiput and/or atlas. The vertebral column is abnormally high and prolapsed into the skull base. As in this case, the odontoid process may compress the cervicomedullary junction. Basilar impression is not synonymous with basilar invagination; basilar impression is reserved for acquired or secondary forms of prolapse, as may occur in patients with Paget's disease, hyperparathyroidism, osteogenesis imperfecta, Hurler's syndrome, and rickets. Platybasia is not synonymous with basilar impression or invagination; platybasia refers to flattening of the skull base, which is manifested as an increase in the Welcker basal angle (the angle formed by the intersection of the nasion-tuberculum and tuberculum-basion lines) above the normal limit of 143°. In the case shown, the Welcker angle cannot be accurately determined because the nasion is not shown; however, the clivus does not appear to have the horizontal orientation usually associated with an increased Welcker angle. The Wackenheim clivus baseline, though, is clearly abnormal. The Wackenheim line is a line along the dorsal surface of the clivus extrapolated into the upper cervical canal. Normally, the Wackenheim line forms a tangent with the posterior aspect of the odontoid tip, but such an arrangement is not observed in this case. The intersection of the Wackenheim line with a line along the posterior body and odontoid process of the axis produces an angle that ranges from 150° in flexion to 180° in extension. The underlying abnormality responsible for basilar invagination in this case involves atlantooccipital assimilation posteriorly given the elongated configuration of the posterior margin of the foramen magnum and lack of a discrete posterior arch of the atlas on the sagittal images. Anteriorly, a malformation involving the atlas and/or proatlas is present.

Notes

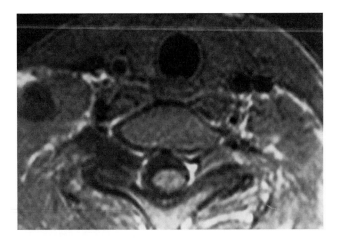
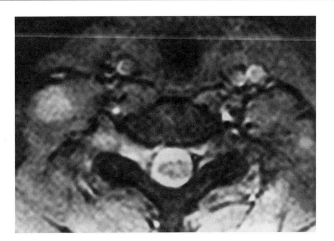

1. Why is this defect unlikely to be a perineurial cyst?

2. What is the likely etiology of the abnormal findings on this T1-weighted image at the level of C7-T1?

3. Does the finding represent nerve root avulsion?

4. What other MR study may be of value in this patient with C7, C8, and T1 abnormalities on electromyographic studies?

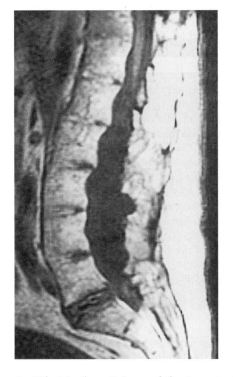
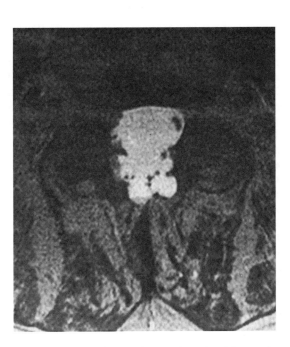

1. What is the etiology of the "empty thecal sac" sign? What is the etiology in this case?

2. Name three congenital conditions associated with dural ectasia.

3. List the three basic types of spinal meningeal cyst.

4. What imaging study would be most useful in diagnosis?

Intramedullary Metastasis (Breast Carcinoma)

1. The enhancement is central rather than peripheral (white matter) within the cord. The corresponding signal intensity on the T2-weighted image is mixed with hyperintense and hypointense areas. The high signal intensity above and below the lesion is also centrally located and extends over a long distance (six vertebral levels); this feature along with cord enlargement suggests edema.

2. Intracranial ependymomas, by about 2:1.

3. Hematogenous spread, because the lesion is located in the center of the cord.

4. False. The thoracic cord is the more common site, most likely because it is longer.

References

Connolly ES Jr, Winfree CJ, McCormick PC, Cruz M, Stein BM: Intramedullary spinal cord metastasis: Report of three cases and review of the literature. *Surg Neurol* 46:329–337, 1996.

Shibamoto Y, Asato R, Abe M: Spinal metastasis from occult intracranial germinoma mimicking primary intramedullary tumour. *Neuroradiology* 36:137–138, 1994.

Cross-Reference

Neuroradiology: THE REQUISITES, pp 487–489.

Comment

Intramedullary metastases are rare. Those resulting from hematogenous spread to the cord cause relatively localized cord enlargement, as opposed to the more diffuse enlargement resulting from contiguous spread of leptomeningeal tumor. Postcontrast T1-weighted images typically show a well-margin-ated, oval enhancing focus, whereas pial metastases are seen as a thin rim of enhancement along the cord surface, with or without nodularity. As illustrated by the T2-weighted image in this case, part or all of the intramedullary lesion may be isointense relative to cord and flanked by high-signal edema. Ependymoma may have a similar appearance. The most common non-CNS malignancies to have intramedullary metastases are breast and lung carcinoma. For 2% of patients with cord metastases, this involvement is the first manifestation of a non-CNS tumor. A few cases of primary brain neoplasm (germinoma, medulloblastoma) metastasizing to the spinal cord, possibly via the central canal of the cord, have been reported.

Notes

Disk Herniation, Thoracic*

1. Focality is generally used to characterize a herniated disk.

2. Below, with T10-11 and T11-12 being the most common levels.

3. The enhancement is due to granulation or scar tissue.

4. Central hypointensity anterior to an inflamed, enhancing posterior longitudinal ligament. Congested epidural veins appearing as triangular areas of enhancement above and below the disk.

References

Parizel PM, Baleriaux D, Rodesch G, et al: Gd-DTPA–enhanced MR in thoracic disc herniations. *Neuroradiology* 31: 75–79, 1989.

Ross JS, Modic MT, Masaryk TJ, et al: Assessment of extradural degenerative disease with Gd-DTPA–enhanced MR imaging: Correlation with surgical and pathologic findings. *AJNR Am J Neuroradiol* 10:1243–1249, 1989.

Cross-Reference

Neuroradiology: THE REQUISITES, pp 461–464.

Comment

Most thoracic disk herniations occur in the lower half of the thoracic spine, as illustrated by this T8-9 right-sided lesion. With spin-echo MR, herniated thoracic disks tend to be isointense to slightly hypointense on T1-weighted images and hypointense on T2-weighted images. Hypointensity reflects disk degeneration with dehydration, or alternatively, calcification. In standard MR imaging protocols for thoracic degenerative disk disease, T1- and T2-weighted sagittal scans are usually accompanied by a gradient-recalled-echo, T2*-weighted axial scan. The latter is particularly sensitive in detecting small extradural defects (noncalcified or calcified herniated disks or osteophytes) indenting the uniformly hyperintense subarachnoid space. One must remember, however, that T2*-weighted images with long echo time (TE) values are very sensitive to susceptibility effects and may exaggerate the size of a small osteophyte or calcified lesion. Gadolinium chelate contrast agents have been used to improve detection of thoracic disk herniations on T1-weighted images based on the findings described above. Herniations, especially chronic ones, sometimes have associated granulation or scar tissue that enhances. This tissue appears to be part of the normal reparative process.

---

*Figures for Case 76 from Madsen PW III, Bowen BC: Spinal cord disease. In: Kelley RE, Ed: *Functional Neuroimaging.* Armonk, NY, Futura, 1994.

Notes

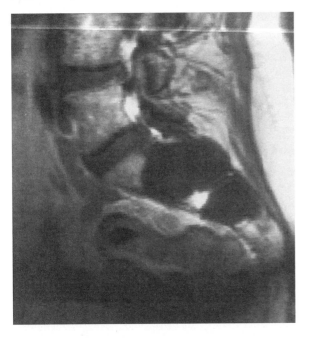

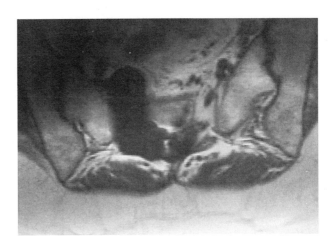

1. Name two types of spinal meningeal cysts.

2. What is Currarino's triad?

3. From what spinal structure does a Tarlov cyst originate?

4. True or false: Most Tarlov cysts are symptomatic.

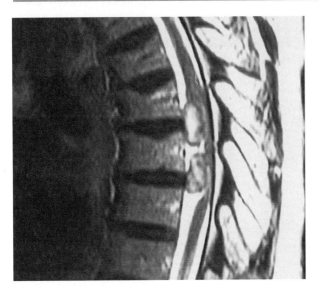

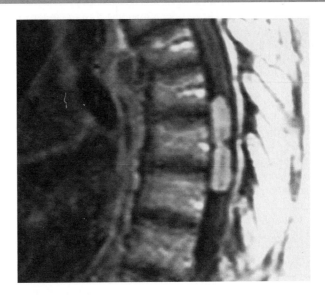

1. What is the most frequent type of intraspinal extramedullary tumor?

2. Are meningiomas and schwannomas strictly extramedullary lesions?

3. Which are more frequently cystic—schwannomas or neurofibromas?

4. Do schwannomas usually arise from motor or sensory roots?

Anterior Sacral Meningocele

1. Extradural cyst without nerve root fibers (type I) and extradural cyst with nerve root fibers (type II).

2. Anorectal malformation, bony sacral defect, and presacral mass.

3. Tarlov perineurial cysts are diverticula of spinal nerve root sleeves.

4. False, although some Tarlov cysts can produce radiculopathy, as well as bowel and bladder dysfunction.

References

Lee SC, Chun YS, Jung SE, Park KW, Kim WK: Currarino triad: Anorectal malformation, sacral bony abnormality, and presacral mass—a review of 11 cases. *J Pediatr Surg* 32:58-61, 1997.

Nabors MW, Pait TG, Byrd EB, et al: Updated assessment and current classification of spinal meningeal cysts. *J Neurosurg* 68:366-377, 1988.

Cross-Reference

Neuroradiology: THE REQUISITES, p 484.

Comment

Classification of spinal meningeal cysts is based on operative inspection and histologic examination, and differentiation between types I and II is difficult on MR imaging. Meningeal cysts are diverticula of the dural sac, nerve root sheath, or arachnoid. All are probably congenital and do, or did at one time, communicate with the subarachnoid space. Type I has a pathologically identifiable pedicle connecting it to the dural sac at the entrance of the dorsal root into the neural foramen (IA, thoracolumbar cyst) or at the caudal tip of the dural sac (IB, sacral meningocele). Type II is a dilatation of the nerve root sleeve; it thus lacks a pedicle and has nerve roots centrally within the cyst or cyst wall. Type II cysts are most often found in the sacrum (Tarlov cysts). Type III cysts are usually located posterior to the cord and may be multiple. Meningeal cysts may enlarge and erode bone, causing foraminal or canal enlargement, or scalloping of the vertebral body.

An anterior sacral meningocele is a herniation of meninges through a congenital defect in the sacrum, coccyx, or adjacent disk spaces in which a CSF-filled mass is formed in the pelvis. The meningocele may occur as an isolated defect; as a manifestation of neurofibromatosis, Marfan syndrome, or other mesenchymal dysplasia; or as part of the syndrome of caudal regression. The defect in the sacrum may be central or paracentral. Its size may vary from barely detectable to extensive, with involvement of one or multiple adjacent foramina (as in this case). The hernia sac may protrude just beyond the surface of the sacrum, as shown on the axial T1-weighted image, or may nearly fill the pelvis. Anterior sacral meningocele is in the differential diagnosis of presacral masses that may be found in Currarino's triad, and consequently, MR imaging is recommended in the workup of these patients to assess the spinal canal and its contents.

Notes

Intradural Schwannoma, Thoracic

1. Schwannoma—29% of cases, versus 25% for meningioma.

2. A few cases of intramedullary schwannoma have been reported. The tumor is thought to arise from peripheral nerves accompanying sulcocommissural branches of the anterior spinal artery into the cord, from developmental inclusion of neural crest cells, or alternatively by ingrowth of tumor from the dorsal root ganglion.

3. Schwannomas.

4. Sensory roots.

Reference

Masaryk TJ: Neoplastic disease of the spine. *Radiol Clin North Am* 29:829-845, 1991.

Cross-Reference

Neuroradiology: THE REQUISITES, pp 489-490.

Comment

Intraspinal schwannomas are usually intradural extramedullary solitary lesions that occur most often in the cervical and thoracic spine, in males, and in the fifth decade of life. They are well encapsulated and composed of Antoni type A and type B tissue, with the latter becoming prominent in larger lesions and being responsible for cyst formation. Larger lesions may appear lobulated and have areas of intrinsic hemorrhage. As shown in this case, schwannomas are typically hyperintense on T2-weighted images and demonstrate enhancement with intravenous gadolinium on T1-weighted images. Two thirds of intraspinal schwannomas are purely intradural, and the remaining third are purely extradural or both intradural and extradural. Schwannoma and neurofibroma may have identical imaging findings. Diffuse, multinodular lesions, referred to as plexiform neurofibromas, are usually associated with neurofibromatosis type 1.

Notes

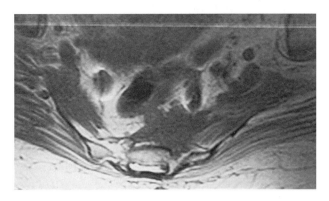
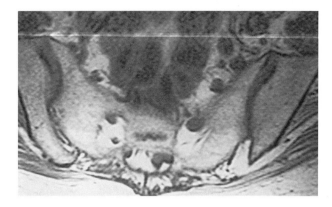

1. Based on these T1-weighted axial images, is this individual more likely to have radiculopathy or plexopathy?

2. The sacral plexus is located on the anterior surface of which muscle?

3. Which of the three connective tissue sheaths within a peripheral nerve is the most impermeable to invasive lesions?

4. List the three pelvic neoplasms that most commonly cause sacral plexopathy.

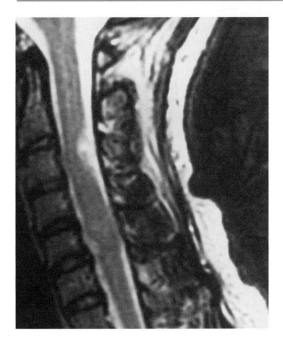
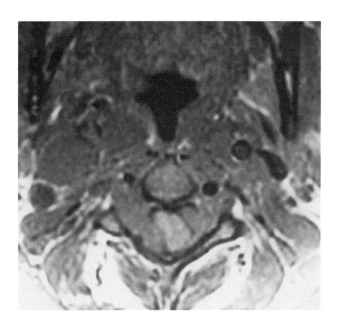

1. Name three neoplasms that may produce the findings observed on the T2-weighted sagittal and the T1-weighted axial (C2-3 level) images.

2. Name three findings, not shown here, that can narrow this differential diagnosis.

3. In this patient, is an intramedullary neoplasm more likely to be an ependymoma or astrocytoma?

4. How might this patient's symptoms differ from those of most patients with the same disorder?

C A S E 7 9

Perineural Spread of Rectosigmoid Carcinoma Along Sacral Nerves*

1. Plexopathy.

2. Piriformis.

3. Perineurium.

4. Colorectal carcinoma, uterine carcinoma, and ovarian carcinoma.

Reference

Pema PJ, Bennett WF, Bova JG, Warman P: CT vs MRI in diagnosis of recurrent rectosigmoid carcinoma. *J Comput Assist Tomogr* 18:256–261, 1994.

Cross-Reference

Neuroradiology: THE REQUISITES, p 491.

Comment

In this case of recurrent rectosigmoid carcinoma after abdominal perineal resection, the axial T1-weighted image at the level of the S4 vertebra *(left image)* demonstrates an infiltrating presacral mass extending from the rectosigmoid region to the anterior surface of the sacrum, which is eroded. The mass is confluent with the left piriformis muscle. At the level of the S3 vertebra *(right image)*, there is relative enlargement of all the nerves that contribute to the left sacral plexus. From a posterior-medial to anterior-lateral direction these nerves are S3 (in the sacral canal), S2, S1, and the lumbosacral trunk (along the anterior surface of the sacrum). Tumor infiltration and retrograde spread along the nerves account for their diffuse enlargement and epidural extension from S2 through S4. When compared with CT, MR imaging has higher sensitivity, specificity, and accuracy in diagnosing recurrent rectosigmoid carcinoma and provides better definition of the extent of tumor.

Consistent with the MR imaging findings in this case, the patient had pain, weakness, and sensory loss in the left leg and foot extending outside the territory of a single root or peripheral nerve. Peripheral nerves have three connective tissue sheaths: endoneurium, perineurium, and epineurium. Perineurium, which consists of dense connective tissue with tight junctions between epithelial-like cells, provides the greatest barrier to axonal damage from neoplasm, infection, or toxic agents.

---

*Figures for Case 79 from Bowen BC: Lumbosacral plexus. In: Stark DD, Bradley WG Jr, Eds: *Magnetic Resonance Imaging*, third edition, Vol 3. Philadelphia, Mosby–Year Book, 1998, pp 1907–1916.

Notes

C A S E 8 0

Neurofibromatosis Type 1, With Cord Compression

1. Nerve sheath tumor (neurofibroma, schwannoma), lymphoma, and metastatic carcinoma.

2. The presence of scoliosis, dural ectasia (lateral meningoceles and scalloping of the posterior margin of the vertebral bodies), and multiple subcutaneous nodules favors neurofibromatosis type 1 (NF1).

3. Astrocytoma.

4. Myelopathy, in addition to the typical clinical findings of pain and radiculopathy associated with spinal nerve sheath tumors.

Reference

Egelhoff JC, Bates DJ, Ross JS, Rothner AD, Cohen BH: Spinal MR findings in neurofibromatosis types 1 and 2. *AJNR Am J Neuroradiol* 13:1071–1077, 1992.

Cross-Reference

Neuroradiology: THE REQUISITES, pp 266–267, 489–490.

Comment

Although the differential diagnosis of bilateral extradural and intradural masses compressing the spinal cord includes both malignant (lymphoma, metastatic carcinoma) and benign (neurofibroma, schwannoma) etiologies, the lack of vertebral destruction on T1- and T2-weighted images favors a benign etiology in a patient with NF1. Neurofibromas consist of both Schwann cells and fibroblasts, arise as a fusiform mass along dorsal sensory nerve rootlets, and are seen in association with NF1. The patient has an increased risk of malignant degeneration in comparison to patients with NF2, for which the principal neoplasms are schwannomas consisting solely of Schwann cells. Malignant nerve sheath tumors develop in 2% to 12% of neurofibromatosis patients and herald a poor prognosis (15% to 30% survival rate at 5 years). NF1 is an autosomal dominant disorder with the genetic mutation located on chromosome 17, whereas chromosome 22 is the site of the mutation in NF2. Associated intramedullary lesions are astrocytomas and "hamartomas" in NF1 and ependymomas in NF2.

Notes

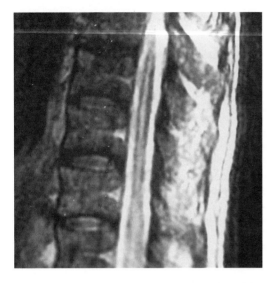
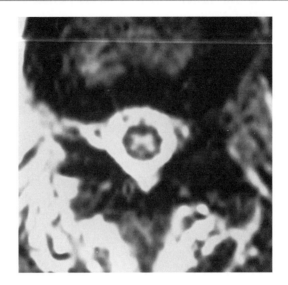

1. Which infectious agents can produce T2 signal abnormalities involving primarily the central gray matter?

2. In cases of spinal cord infarction, what extramedullary MR imaging findings have been reported?

3. Where do cord infarcts occur most commonly?

4. How does the pattern of hyperintensity shown on the axial T2-weighted image differ from that associated with amyotrophic lateral sclerosis (ALS)?

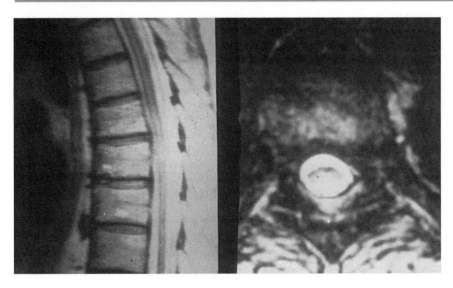

1. What is the most common spinal cord pathology of AIDS patients at autopsy: HIV myelitis, vacuolar myelopathy, or toxoplasmic myelitis?

2. What part of the cord is most severely affected?

3. What disorder of known etiology produces similar pathologic findings?

4. Which is more likely to show a focal lesion on T2-weighted MR imaging: HIV myelitis or vacuolar myelopathy?

CASE 81

Spinal Cord Infarction, Thoracic

1. Poliovirus, coxsackievirus, and other enteroviruses.

2. Abnormal signal within a vertebral body that is supplied by the same segmental artery as the affected region of the cord. Absence of a "flow void" in the distal aorta as a result of occlusion may also be detected.

3. Thoracolumbar region.

4. In this case the central gray matter is hyperintense. In ALS, hyperintense signal, when present, usually involves the white matter of the lateral corticospinal tracts symmetrically.

References

Haddad MC, Al-Thagafi MYA, Djurberg H: MRI of spinal cord and vertebral body infarction in the anterior spinal artery syndrome. *Neuroradiology* 38:161-162, 1996.

Yuh WTC, Marsh EE, Wang AK, et al: MR imaging of spinal cord and vertebral body infarction. *AJNR Am J Neuroradiol* 13:145-154, 1992.

Cross-Reference

Neuroradiology: THE REQUISITES, pp 495-496.

Comment

On T2-weighted MR images, cord infarction is detected as a short or long segment of increased signal intensity primarily involving the central gray matter. In the acute/subacute stage, this increased intensity represents edema, and the cord is usually enlarged. When infarction results from compromise of a segmental artery, branches supplying the ipsilateral half of the vertebral body may also be affected. A vertebral body infarct is best detected on sagittal images, where it usually appears as a triangular area of increased signal near the end-plate and/or deep medullary portion of the vertebral body. When cord and vertebral body signal abnormalities involve the same or adjacent spinal segments, segmental artery occlusion should be suspected.

Neurodegenerative diseases that involve the anterior horn cells (ALS and spinal muscular atrophy) can in theory produce T2 prolongation in the central gray matter, although cord signal abnormalities in patients with ALS are typically located in the lateral corticospinal tracts and no postcontrast enhancement is seen. The clinical history in ALS (gradual onset, fasciculations, muscle weakness and wasting without sensory loss) also differs from that of cord infarction (abrupt onset, anterior spinal artery syndrome).

Notes

CASE 82

Vacuolar Myelopathy

1. Vacuolar myelopathy.

2. Lateral and posterior columns of the thoracic cord.

3. Subacute combined degeneration caused by vitamin B_{12} deficiency or, uncommonly, folic acid deficiency.

4. HIV myelitis.

References

Petito CK: The neuropathology of human immunodeficiency virus infection of the spinal cord. In: Berger JR, Levy RM, Eds: *AIDS and the Nervous System,* second edition. Philadelphia, Lippincott-Raven, 1997, pp 451-459.

Quencer RM, Post MJ: Spinal cord lesions in patients with AIDS. *Neuroimaging Clin N Am* 7:359-373, 1997.

Cross-Reference

Neuroradiology: THE REQUISITES, p 480.

Comment

The T2-weighted images show a nonenlarged cord with diffuse hyperintensity in the lower thoracic region. On the axial image, the anterior portion of the cord appears relatively spared in this proven case of vacuolar myelopathy. In such instances, light and electron microscopy reveal vacuolation in the white matter of the spinal cord in association with lipid-laden macrophages. Demyelination and inflammation are typically absent. The pathologic changes tend to be symmetrically distributed; they involve the white matter diffusely yet favor the lateral and posterior columns. The pathologic findings in HIV myelitis differ from those in vacuolar myelopathy in that involvement is more focal, microglial nodules and multinuclear giant cells are found in the gray matter (and sometimes white matter), and white matter lesions with inflammation are present. On T2-weighted images, then, one may expect more focal hyperintensity in cases of HIV myelitis than in vacuolar myelopathy. On postcontrast T1-weighted images, cord enhancement is absent in vacuolar myelopathy and occurs only rarely in cases of HIV myelitis. Both lesions, as well as progressive multifocal leukoencephalopathy, should be included in the differential diagnosis of an abnormal cord signal without a mass effect or cord enlargement in an AIDS patient.

Petito reviewed five neuropathologic series from the literature and found that the frequency of various spinal cord diseases in adult AIDS patients was as follows:

1. Vacuolar myelopathy, 14% to 54%

2. HIV myelitis, 5% to 8%

3. Opportunistic infection, 8% to 15% (including cytomegalovirus, 3% to 8%; herpes simplex virus, 2%; varicella-zoster virus, 1%; fungal infection, 4%; bacterial infection, 2%; and toxoplasmosis, 1%)

4. Nonspecific myelitis, 7% to 36%

5. Lymphoma, 2% to 8%

6. Others, 1% to 8%

Many patients had more than one of the diseases listed above. In approximately 50% to 60% of the patients, the spinal cord was normal.

Notes

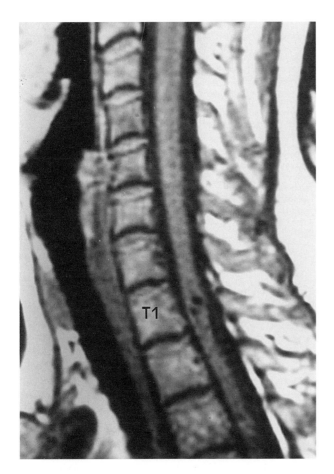 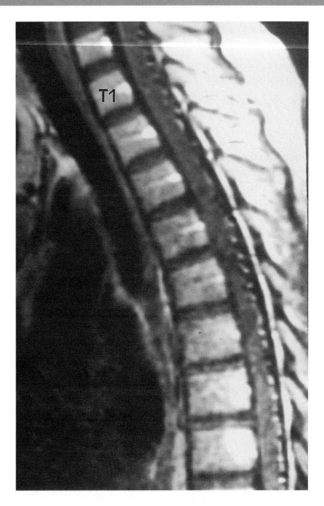

1. Name three causes of marked hypointensity in the cord on T1- and T2-weighted images.

2. How do you explain the intramedullary enhancement in the postcontrast T1-weighted image?

3. Which of the following is most likely to be manifested as subarachnoid hemorrhage: dural arteriovenous (AV) fistula, intramedullary AV malformation (AVM), or cavernous angioma?

4. Name two pathways for blood flow between the veins on the anterior and posterior surfaces of the cord.

Intramedullary Arteriovenous Malformation (T1)

1. Blood flow, calcification, and chronic hemorrhage (hemosiderin/ferritin).

2. Venous hypertension with or without venous infarction.

3. Intramedullary AVM.

4. The coronal (or perimedullary) venous plexus surrounding the cord and transmedullary anastomoses connecting the anterior and posterior median veins directly.

Reference

Berenstein A, Lasjaunias P: Endovascular treatment of spine and spinal cord lesions. In: Lasjaunias P, Berenstein P, Eds: *Surgical Neuroangiography*, Vol 5. New York, Springer-Verlag, 1992, pp 1–47.

Cross-Reference

Neuroradiology: THE REQUISITES, pp 496–497.

Comment

The precontrast T1-weighted image demonstrates a focal low-signal intensity lesion within the cord at the T1 level with subtle scalloping of the posterior cord surface immediately inferior to the lesion. The postcontrast image (upper thoracic spine) shows serpentine enhancement along the posterior surface of the cord and diffuse enhancement within the cord inferior to T6. No significant cord enlargement is seen, and the lesion at the T1 level has subtle hypointensity mixed with mild enhancement on the postcontrast image. These findings are explained by the presence of a glomus AVM at T1. Glomus (type II) AVMs are intramedullary in location and have a compact nidus. They are high-flow vascular malformations capable of producing flow voids on precontrast spin-echo images. Drainage into the coronal venous plexus on the cord surface, with engorgement of the posterior and/or anterior median vein, results in a variable appearance of perimedullary flow voids and cord scalloping on precontrast images, as well as serpentine enhancement on postcontrast images. Venous hypertension resulting from AVM drainage can impede venous drainage from normal areas of the cord at a distance from the lesion. These areas, such as the lower thoracic cord in this case, may then show enhancement as a result of persistence of gadolinium within intramedullary veins and venules. With chronic venous congestion, venous infarction and breakdown of the blood-cord barrier may ensue, also contributing to cord enhancement. This same mechanism explains cord enhancement from dural AV fistulas (type I spinal AVMs).

Notes

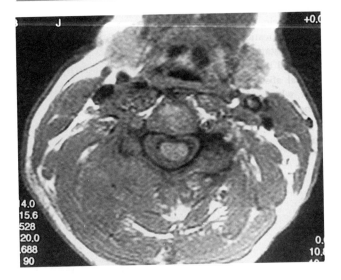

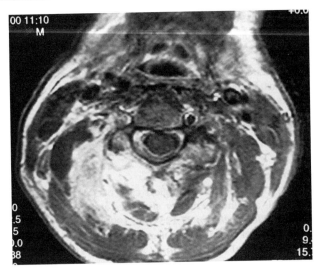

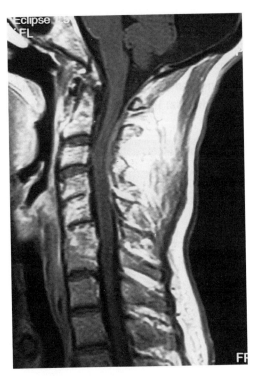

1. Name three conditions that would predispose this patient to the abnormalities shown on the precontrast and postcontrast axial (C3-4 level) and the postcontrast sagittal T1-weighted images.

2. What paraspinal muscle groups are primarily involved?

3. What is the most common organism responsible for vertebral osteomyelitis? for spinal epidural abscess?

4. What is the most common location for spinal epidural abscess—the cervical, thoracic, or lumbar spine?

Neuroblastoma

1. Neuroblastoma, rhabdomyosarcoma, and peripheral primitive neuroectodermal tumor (PPNET).

2. The patient is a 3-year-old boy with extensive tumor. The differential diagnosis for neuroblastoma, which occurs primarily in children younger than 5 years, includes ganglioneuroblastoma and ganglio-neuroma, which are usually seen in children between 5 and 8 years of age.

3. Approximately 14% of patients with neuroblastoma or ganglioneuroblastoma have intraspinal extension of their tumor based on surgical data.

4. Neuroblastoma and other neuroectodermal tumors may arise from primordia of the intraspinal posterior root ganglion.

References

Siegel MJ, Jamroz GA, Glazer HS, Abramson CL: MR imaging of intraspinal extension of neuroblastoma. *J Comput Assist Tomogr* 10:593–595, 1986.

Smith EI, Castleberry RP: Neuroblastoma. *Curr Probl Surg* 27:573–620, 1990.

Cross-Reference

Neuroradiology: THE REQUISITES, p 493.

Comment

Among the tumors derived from primitive neural crest cells are PPNETs, neuroblastomas, ganglioneuroblastomas, and ganglioneuromas. They can originate in the adrenal medulla or paravertebral sympathetic chain. Histologically, neuroblastomas and PPNETs are among the group of small blue round cell tumors, which include rhabdomyosarcoma, Ewing's sarcoma, extranodal lymphoma of soft tissue, and small cell osteogenic sarcoma.

In order of cellular differentiation, ganglioneuroblastoma is intermediate between neuroblastoma and ganglioneuroma, which consists almost entirely of mature ganglion cells. From their usual thoracic or lumbar paravertebral location, these tumors can extend into the spinal canal via the neural foramina and produce the "dumbbell" appearance shown on the axial (L4-5 level) image. MR signal intensity and enhancement may be relatively uniform, as in this case, or variable, especially when cystic or hemorrhagic necrosis is present. In the cervical region, intraspinal extension of tumor is rare.

Notes

Adult Tethered Cord With a Dermal Sinus

1. The patient's symptoms are probably due to a congenitally tethered cord and were precipitated by trauma, which also caused a burst fracture of L4.

2. Does the patient have any of the cutaneous manifestations associated with spinal dysraphism—midline dimple or ostium, palpable cord-like tract, local hyperpigmentation, hairy nevus, or capillary angioma?

3. Based on the axial T1-weighted image, one should question whether a dermal sinus tract is present. If so, it is possible for bacteria on the skin to infect the subarachnoid space.

4. When it is greater than 2 mm in diameter.

Reference

Yamada S, Iacono RP, Andrade T, Mandybur G, Yamada BS: Pathophysiology of tethered cord syndrome. *Neurosurg Clin N Am* 6:311–323, 1995.

Cross-Reference

Neuroradiology: THE REQUISITES, pp 482–484.

Comment

Tethered cord syndrome, manifested by motor and sensory dysfunction and incontinence, is caused by excessive tension in the lumbosacral cord. The underlying mechanism is related to impairment of oxidative metabolism in this region. The symptoms of adult tethered cord are more often seen in young women than in men and are often precipitated by a traumatic event. As shown here, the conus is usually low lying (below L2), although distinction between this structure and a thickened filum may be difficult. The finding of a bony defect in the sacral region with intervening fat at S1 on the sagittal image is consistent with lipomyeloschisis or a dorsal dermal sinus surrounded by fat. The latter is suggested by the findings on the axial T1-weighted image at the S1 level, which shows a midline hypointense band outlined by hyperintense fat.

Notes

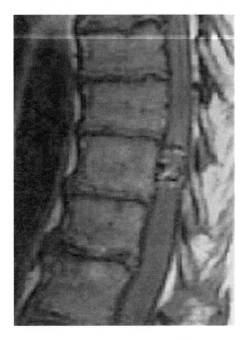
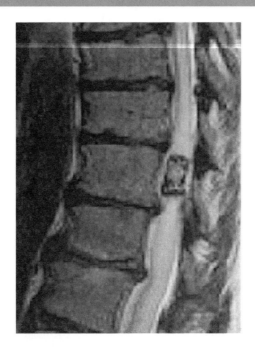

1. List four nontraumatic causes of hematomyelia.

2. In addition to the T1- and T2-weighted spin-echo images shown here, what additional MR imaging studies may help differentiate one cause from another?

3. What is the most common calcified intramedullary tumor?

4. Should the lesion shown in this case be resected?

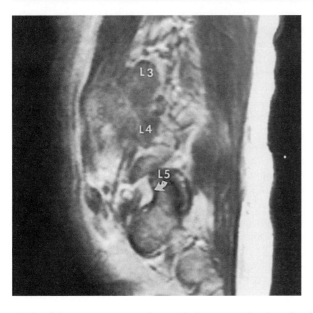
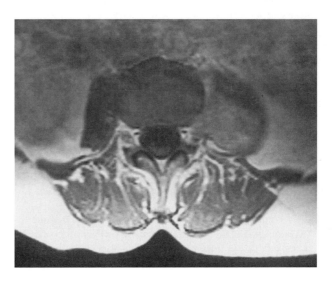

1. In this case you are shown left parasagittal and axial (L3-4 level) postcontrast T1-weighted images. Where is the lumbar plexus located?

2. Which has a higher rate of malignant change, schwannoma or plexiform neurofibroma?

3. Are areas of hemorrhage more commonly seen in schwannomas or in plexiform neurofibromas?

4. What distinguishes benign and malignant nerve sheath tumors on MR imaging?

Cavernous Angioma

1. Intramedullary arteriovenous malformation (AVM), cavernous angioma, ependymoma, and hemangioblastoma.

2. Gradient-echo MR imaging with a relatively long echo time (TE), postcontrast T1-weighted images and MR angiography, and MR imaging of the brain.

3. Astrocytoma.

4. A cavernous malformation can be resected or merely observed, depending on its evolution, location, and surgical accessibility.

References

Dillon WJ: Cryptic vascular malformations: Controversies in terminology, diagnosis, pathophysiology, and treatment. *AJNR Am J Neuroradiol* 18:1839–1846, 1997.

Turjman F, Joly D, Monnet O, Faure C, Doyon D, Froment JC: MRI of intramedullary cavernous haemangiomas. *Neuroradiology* 37:297–302, 1995.

Cross-Reference

Neuroradiology: THE REQUISITES, pp 496–498.

Comment

Intramedullary and intracranial cavernous angiomas have a similar appearance on MR imaging—heterogeneous signal intensity (from accumulations of blood products of varying age) on both T1- and T2-weighted MR images, with a surrounding rim of hypointensity (primarily from hemosiderin) on T2-weighted images. Intramedullary lesions with an extramedullary component and lesions with associated syringomyelia have been described. On gradient-echo T2*-weighted images, hypointense zones comprising these lesions appear much larger. This feature differentiates hypointensity caused by hemosiderin and/or calcification from that caused by flowing blood ("flow void" associated with AVM) and increases the sensitivity of MR imaging in detecting cavernous angiomas. The cord may or may not be enlarged by these lesions. Spinal x-ray angiographic findings are normal, and postcontrast MR angiography shows normal intradural veins. Progressive myelopathy is the most frequent clinical finding.

Cavernous angiomas are the most common form of cryptic vascular malformation, for which the risk of hemorrhage is between 0.25% and 0.7% per year (increasing to 4.5% in patients with a previous clinical hemorrhage). Surgical resection (which was the method of treatment in this case) is generally recommended for patients with symptomatic hemorrhage. When spinal MR imaging reveals a probable cryptic vascular malformation, imaging of the brain is recommended because of the familial occurrence of multiple cavernous angiomas involving the brain and spinal cord. In most cases, though, cavernous angiomas are sporadic and are thought to represent an acquired disease of venous origin rather than a true developmental malformation of blood vessels.

Notes

Malignant Peripheral Nerve Sheath Tumor*

1. In the psoas muscle.

2. Plexiform neurofibroma.

3. Schwannoma.

4. Many studies indicate that benign and malignant nerve sheath tumors can be indistinguishable, particularly when large; however, in one study the "target sign" was found to reliably discriminate between benign (benign neurofibroma) and malignant tumors.

Reference

Bhargava R, Parham DM, Lasater OE, Chari RS, Chen G, Fletcher BD: MR imaging differentiation of benign and malignant peripheral nerve sheath tumors: Use of the target sign. *Pediatr Radiol* 27:124–129, 1997.

Cross-Reference

Neuroradiology: THE REQUISITES, pp 267.

Comment

Because most malignant tumors derived from the nerve sheath have immunohistochemical profiles that share features of both schwannomas and neurofibromas, the designation "malignant peripheral nerve sheath tumor" (MPNST) is now used in place of terms such as "malignant schwannoma" and "neurofibrosarcoma." Malignant degeneration of nerve sheath tumors is uncommon. It occurs in about 5% (a range of 2% to 13% is sometimes cited) of cases of neurofibromatosis type 1 (NF1) and is rarely seen in cases of NF2 with multiple schwannomas.

The imaging features of benign and malignant nerve sheath tumors overlap with respect to size, margin sharpness, heterogeneity of signal intensity, contrast enhancement, and corresponding muscle atrophy. One finding that has been described for benign neurofibroma but is lacking in MPNST is a central hypointensity with peripheral hyperintensity on T2-weighted images, called the "target sign." Histologically, the central area consists of a variable mixture of cellular elements and collagen, whereas the periphery is myxoid tissue. One study found that the sensitivity of the target sign for benign neurofibroma was 100% and the specificity, 92%. The lesion involving the L3 and L4 nerves in this case had inhomogeneous signal on T2-weighted images without a target sign, and on the postcontrast T1-weighted images (shown here) it appeared to infiltrate the left psoas muscle.

---

*Figures for Case 90 from Bowen BC: Lumbosacral plexus. In: Stark DD, Bradley WG Jr, Eds: *Magnetic Resonance Imaging*, third edition, Vol 3. Philadelphia, Mosby–Year Book, 1998, pp 1907–1916.

Notes

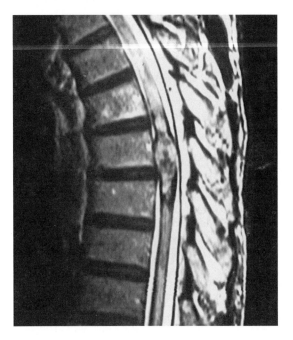 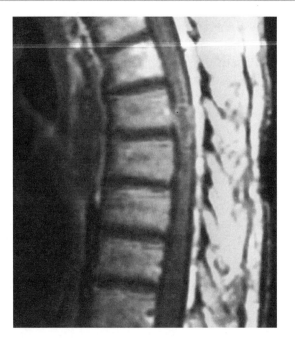

1. Is the lesion at T6-7 shown above (T2-weighted and postcontrast T1-weighted images) more likely to be an astrocytoma, a hemangioblastoma, or an ependymoma?

2. Name three intramedullary lesions that have been shown to cause superficial siderosis of the CNS.

3. Is intramedullary ependymoma more likely to cause symmetric or asymmetric enlargement of the cord?

4. Name three intramedullary lesions that tend to have associated nonenhancing cysts.

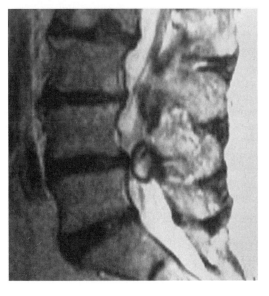 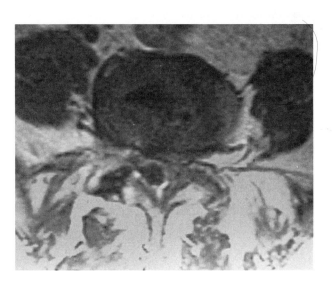

1. What is the differential diagnosis for the findings on the T2-weighted FSE (fast-spin-echo) sagittal and postcontrast T1-weighted axial images?

2. What is the likely etiology of this lesion?

3. At what spinal level is it most commonly found?

4. How might you explain a sudden exacerbation of chronic back pain in this patient?

Ependymoma, Thoracic

1. Ependymoma, because there is evidence of focal, rather than diffuse, cord enlargement as well as hemorrhage.

2. Arteriovenous malformation, ependymoma, and hemangioblastoma.

3. Symmetric, because the tumor arises from ependymal cells in the central canal.

4. Ependymoma, hemangioblastoma, and astrocytoma.

Reference

Kahan H, Sklar EM, Post MJ, Bruce JH: MR characteristics of histopathologic subtypes of spinal ependymoma. *AJNR Am J Neuroradiol* 17:143–150, 1996.

Cross-Reference

Neuroradiology: THE REQUISITES, pp 486–487.

Comment

Ependymomas account for 40% to 60% of primary spinal cord tumors, and about 60% of ependymomas occur in the conus medullaris/cauda equina region. These masses are well-circumscribed, noninfiltrating, benign tumors that are generally more focal than astrocytomas and potentially totally resectable. They have a propensity for intratumoral hemorrhage and may also produce subarachnoid hemorrhage with leptomeningeal deposition of hemosiderin (superficial siderosis). Cystic degeneration of the tumor may be observed, as well as extensive cyst formation rostral and/or caudal to the tumor. Ependymomas in the filum are usually of the myxopapillary histologic subtype. This subtype tends to be hyperintense on precontrast T1-weighted images, whereas most nonmyxopapillary tumors are not. On T2-weighted images, intramedullary tumor, as well as surrounding edema, is hyperintense, although hemorrhage results in central and/or peripheral hypointensity from hemosiderin (as shown above). On postcontrast T1-weighted images, the pattern of enhancement is variable, with homogeneous (38%), heterogeneous (31%), rim-like (19%), minimal (6%), or no (6%) enhancement observed in one series of 26 proven spinal ependymomas.

Notes

Juxtaarticular Cyst, Lumbar

1. Migrated herniated disk, perineurial cyst, cystic schwannoma, and juxtaarticular (synovial or ganglion) cyst.

2. Right facet joint degeneration.

3. L4-5.

4. Hemorrhage within the cyst.

References

Jackson DE Jr, Atlas SW, Mani JR, Norman D: Intraspinal synovial cysts: MR imaging. *Radiology* 170:527–530, 1989.

Liu SS, Williams KD, Drayer BP, Spetzler RF, Sonntag VK: Synovial cysts of the lumbosacral spine: Diagnosis by MR imaging. *AJNR Am J Neuroradiol* 10:1239–1242, 1989.

Cross-Reference

Neuroradiology: THE REQUISITES, p 467.

Comment

Findings that help characterize this intraspinal, juxtaarticular cyst are its location (epidural, posterolateral), its apparent continuity with a hypointense, hypertrophic (degenerated) right facet joint, and its hypointense rim on the T2-weighted image. These cysts may have variable signal intensity, depending on whether they contain synovial or other watery fluid, blood or proteinaceous material, or air. The hypointensity of the rim on T2-weighted images has been attributed to the presence of a fibrous capsule with hemosiderin deposits and/or fine calcification. Postcontrast enhancement of the rim, as seen here, probably reflects the presence of inflammation. Pain with or without radiculopathy is commonly present and may be due to a mass effect of the cyst on the dorsal roots and/or the underlying facet arthritis. Hemorrhage into a cyst has been proposed as a mechanism to explain acute exacerbation of chronic low back pain. On the other hand, spontaneous resolution of symptoms has been attributed to decompression of the cyst into the adjacent facet joint as inflammation resolves.

The other lesions in the differential diagnosis do not have the combination of findings described here. It is rare to find a herniated disk fragment posterior to the thecal sac, and such a fragment is never found posterior to the ligamentum flavum, where juxtaarticular cysts are located. A perineurial cyst is typically associated with the nerve root sleeve in the neural foramen and is separate from the facet joint. Cystic schwannoma is usually an intradural lesion and does not have a hypointense rim. An air-filled cyst may be indistinguishable from an osteophyte on MR imaging, but the two are easily differentiated with CT.

Notes

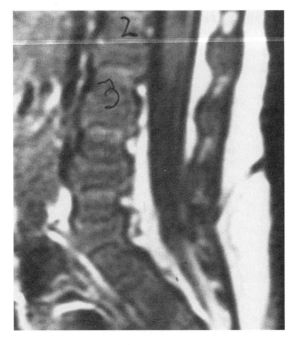
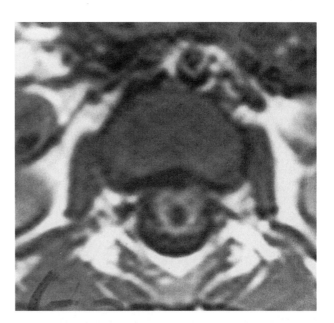

1. Name three entities that may account for the cystic area of the conus in this infant.
2. What is the next most common craniospinal location for the anomaly shown here?
3. Are more or fewer than 50% of patients with this anomaly likely to have a tethered cord?
4. What lumbosacral dysraphic defect is strongly associated with dermoid or epidermoid cyst?

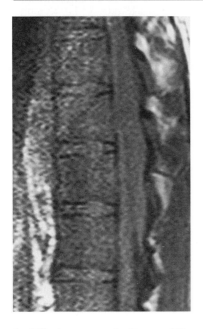
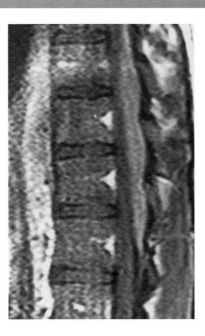

1. What nonneoplastic condition may produce the findings shown on these pre- and postcontrast images?
2. Among neoplastic etiologies, do you favor metastatic disease or hematopoietic malignancy? Why?
3. Would you recommend a myelogram to determine whether a "block" is present?
4. For hematopoietic malignancies, which is more useful to monitor treatment: T1 or T2 relaxation time?

Dermal Sinus Tract

1. Epidermoid/dermoid cyst, terminal syringohydromyelia, and ventriculus terminalis.

2. Occiput.

3. More than 50%.

4. Dorsal dermal sinus.

References

Barkovich AJ, Edwards MS, Cogen PH: MR evaluation of spinal dermal sinus tracts in children. *AJNR Am J Neuroradiol* 12:123–129, 1991.

Iskandar BJ, Oakes WJ, McLaughlin C, Osumi AK, Tien RD: Terminal syringohydromyelia and occult spinal dysraphism. *J Neurosurg* 81:513–519, 1994.

Cross-Reference

Neuroradiology: THE REQUISITES, p 484.

Comment

Dorsal dermal sinus is a midline epithelium-lined tract that extends inward from the skin surface and may terminate in subcutaneous tissue or continue deeper and terminate at the meninges, nerve roots, filum terminale, conus, or cord. The most common location is the sacrococcygeal region, where the sinus rarely communicates with the spinal canal; however, in the lumbosacral region, communication with the canal is more common, and seeding of the tract with bacteria from the skin may result in local abscess, arachnoiditis, and/or meningitis. As shown here, the MR image appearance of a dermal sinus is that of a thin, low–signal intensity band extending through subcutaneous and deeper fat. While the intraspinal portion of the tract may be poorly seen, local outpouching or "beaking" of the thecal sac can be helpful in identifying the junction of the dermal sinus with the dura. In 60% to 80% of cases of lumbosacral dermal sinus, the position of the conus is low, which implies tethering of the spinal cord. In the case shown here, the position of the conus is borderline, being located at L2-3. A sacral dimple and pilonidal sinus may resemble a dermal sinus tract; however, the first two lesions are always near the anus and extend inferiorly or horizontally toward the dorsal surface of the coccyx.

In approximately 50% of cases of dermal sinus, the inner portion of the tract enlarges to form a dermoid or epidermoid cyst. These possibilities must therefore be at the forefront of the differential diagnosis for the cystic area of the conus. Terminal syringohydromyelia, defined as cystic dilatation in the lower third of the spinal cord, is frequently associated with occult spinal dysraphism. Ventriculus terminalis is a normal developmental phenomenon, usually detected incidentally, with a volume (average of 0.18 cm^3) that is less than that observed in cases of syringohydromyelia.

Notes

Acute Myeloid Leukemia With Granulocytic Sarcoma (Chloroma)

1. Extramedullary hematopoiesis.

2. Hematopoietic malignancy, because of the diffuse, homogeneous involvement of the vertebrae and the extensive posterior epidural mass.

3. No, because of the small yet definite possibility of catastrophic myelopathy following lumbar puncture in patients with epidural masses compressing the cord and because the lesion is well characterized by MR imaging.

4. T1 relaxation time has been used to assess the stage (newly diagnosed, relapse, remission) of disease in children with leukemia.

References

Kim JK, Ryu KN, Choi WS, Choe BK, Choi JM, Yoon AY: Spinal involvement of hematopoietic malignancies and metastasis: Differentiation using MR imaging. *Clin Imaging* 23:125–133, 1999.

Wong MC, Krol G, Rosenblum MK: Occult epidural chloroma complicated by acute paraplegia following lumbar puncture. *Ann Neurol* 31:110–112, 1992.

Cross-Reference

Neuroradiology: THE REQUISITES, pp 491–492.

Comment

On the precontrast T1-weighted image of the lower thoracic spine (obtained at 1.0 tesla), the signal intensity of the vertebrae is less than that of the intervertebral disks. This finding is generally abnormal, except in infants and young children, and suggests a process that diffusely affects the vertebral marrow. The postcontrast image shows slight enhancement of the vertebrae (the inhomogeneity is due to artifacts). A prevertebral enhancing mass is present. A homogeneously enhancing posterior epidural mass is compressing the lower thoracic cord in this 25-year-old man with lower extremity dysesthesias. The differential diagnosis includes hematopoietic malignancies (lymphoma, leukemia, multiple myeloma), metastatic disease, and extramedullary hematopoiesis. The findings favor a hematopoietic malignancy, especially in the absence of cortical destruction. Infiltration of vertebral marrow by leukemic cells prolongs the T1 relaxation time and can be used to assess the stage of disease. Although dependent on the field strength of the magnet and the method used to prescribe a region of interest (e.g., avoid the posterior basivertebral vein or cortex), the T1 relaxation time of marrow in pediatric patients with newly diagnosed leukemia has been shown to be approximately twice that of normal individuals and patients in remission.

This patient had acute myeloid leukemia, and the epidural mass proved to be a chloroma, so called because of the greenish color of the fresh specimen. Chloroma occurs in about 3% of patients with myeloid leukemia or myeloproliferative disorders. Less commonly, it may occur in the absence of evidence of systemic disease; however, acute leukemia develops in almost all nonleukemic patients with chloroma within months (average, 10.5 months) of diagnosis. The histogenesis of chloroma of the spine is uncertain, although embryonic nests in the spinal dura mater could be the cells of origin.

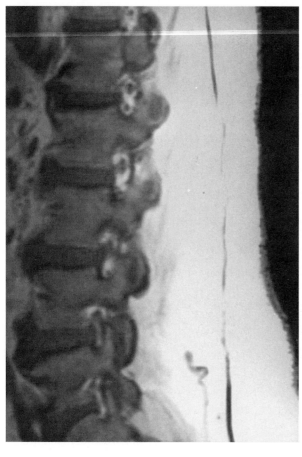

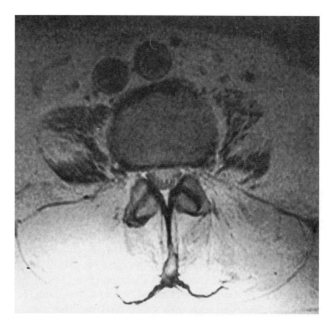

1. Identify the abnormality on the parasagittal T1-weighted image and the axial fast-spin-echo T2-weighted image (L4 level). Name two categories of disorders that may produce this appearance.

2. Could the findings in this 52-year-old man with weakness be due to a lumbar plexus lesion?

3. What structure produces the low–signal intensity stripe identified between the spine and the skin on the parasagittal image?

4. What is "pseudohypertrophy" in the context of this case?

Muscular Dystrophy

1. The erector spinae muscles are nearly absent. Muscular dystrophy and spinal muscular atrophy.

2. No.

3. Fascial sheath of the paraspinous muscle.

4. Enlargement of certain muscle groups, usually the calf muscles, in individuals with Duchenne's muscular dystrophy.

Reference

Murphy WA, Totty WG, Carroll JE: MRI of normal and pathologic skeletal muscle. *AJR Am J Roentgenol* 146:565-574, 1986.

Cross-Reference

Neuroradiology: THE REQUISITES, pp 453-455.

Comment

In this individual with a history of muscular dystrophy, the normal erector spinae muscles are not seen on the parasagittal image. The axial image shows fatty replacement of the psoas muscles and almost complete replacement of the erector spinae muscles. Muscular dystrophy refers to a group of genetically determined myopathies characterized by progressive atrophy or degeneration of increasing numbers of individual muscle cells. Traditionally, muscular dystrophies are subdivided according to the pattern of initial muscle involvement: (1) Duchenne's (X-linked recessive), which involves the pelvic girdle initially; (2) limb girdle (autosomal recessive); and (3) facioscapulohumeral (autosomal recessive), which involves the face and shoulder girdle. The latter two are found in males and females equally, and pseudohypertrophy is not a regular feature. In patients with Duchenne's muscular dystrophy, complete paralysis and death usually ensue within the first two decades of life. This individual has a benign variant of the Duchenne type that may begin as late as the fourth decade and has minimal effect on life span.

The MR findings cannot be due to a lumbar plexus lesion because of involvement of the erector spinae muscles, which are innervated by the dorsal rami of the spinal nerves. The lumbar and sacral plexuses are formed from the ventral rami. The fascial sheath surrounding the erector spinae muscles is more prominent on these images because it is outlined by the fat-replaced muscle and subcutaneous fat.

Notes

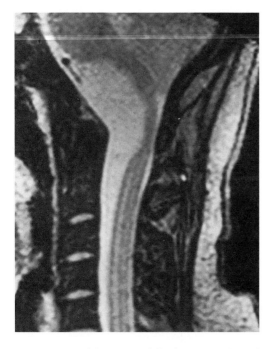
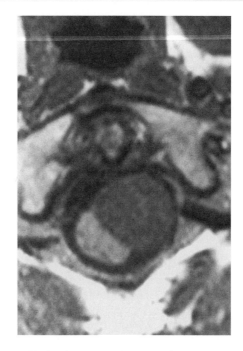

1. How would you modify the sagittal gradient-recalled-echo (GRE) T2*-weighted image to improve contrast between a suspected lesion and CSF?

2. Name three lesions that may cause the abnormalities shown on the T2*- and T1-weighted images above.

3. One of these lesions is strongly associated with congenital anomalies. Name three of the anomalies.

4. This lesion sometimes has high signal on T1- and T2-weighted images. Why?

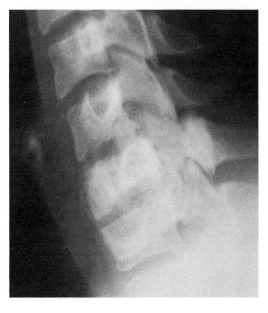
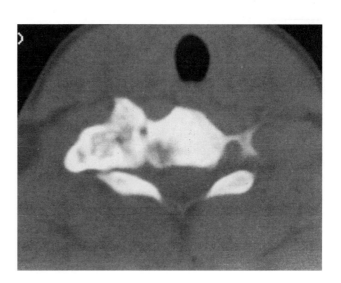

1. Which parts of the vertebra are abnormal?

2. Name at least three causes of "ivory vertebra."

3. How is osteoid osteoma differentiated from osteoblastoma?

4. Do they have the same distribution of occurrence along the spinal axis?

CASE 96

Enterogenous Cyst

1. Vary the flip angle, because this is the primary determinant of contrast on GRE images. By decreasing the flip angle, contrast based on T2 differences will improve.

2. Enterogenous cyst, epidermoid cyst, or arachnoid cyst (containing proteinaceous material).

3. Spina bifida (anterior or posterior), fused vertebrae, and hemivertebrae.

4. The cyst is lined by mucin-secreting cells, so the cyst fluid may be rich in macromolecules. These molecules alter the T1 and T2 relaxation times of the fluid in such a way that the fluid can be hyperintense on both T1- and T2-weighted images. The effect is analogous to that described for mucoceles and chronic secretions in the paranasal sinuses.

Reference

Nalm-ur-Rahman, Jamjoom A, al-Rajeh SM, al-Sohaibani MO: Spinal intradural extramedullary enterogenous cysts. Report of two cases and review of literature. *J Neuroradiol* 21:262–266, 1994.

Cross-Reference

Neuroradiology: THE REQUISITES, p 484.

Comment

The sagittal T2*-weighted image demonstrates subtle differences in signal intensity between the region of cord compression at the craniocervical junction and the CSF in the prepontine cistern and subarachnoid space anterior to the cervical cord. The axial T1-weighted image shows the difference in signal intensity better, so a mass anterior to the cord is easily delineated. The findings are consistent with an intradural, extramedullary cyst-like mass, and congenital, infectious, or neoplastic cystic lesions should be included in the differential diagnosis. An enterogenous (or neurenteric) cyst is relatively rare and identified by the presence of mucin-secreting, columnar epithelium, usually lacking cilia, similar to that of the gastrointestinal tract. The cyst is generally found in the cervical region anterior to the cord in an intradural, extramedullary location. Most patients are younger than 40 years at the time of diagnosis and have a slowly progressive myelopathy. About 50% of patients have other congenital anomalies, such as the vertebral defects noted above and fistulous communications with cysts in the mediastinum, thorax, or abdomen.

Notes

CASE 97

Osteoblastoma, Cervical

1. The vertebral arch, right transverse process, and body.

2. Hodgkin's lymphoma, osteoblastic metastasis, Paget's disease, and osteoblastoma.

3. By the size of the central vascular nidus: smaller than 1.5 cm is osteoid osteoma, larger than 1.5 cm is osteoblastoma.

4. Yes, lumbar > cervical > thoracic.

References

Murphey MD, Andrews CL, Flemming DJ, Temple HT, Smith WS, Smirniotopoulos JG: From the archives of the AFIP. Primary tumors of the spine: Radiologic pathologic correlation. *Radiographics* 16:1131–1158, 1996.

Sherazi Z, Saifuddin A, Shaikh MI, Natali C, Pringle JA: Unusual imaging findings in association with spinal osteoblastoma. *Clin Radiol* 51:644–648, 1996.

Cross-Reference

Neuroradiology: THE REQUISITES, p 494.

Comment

The lateral radiograph of the cervical spine demonstrates sclerosis and thickening in the region of the C6 vertebral body, the overlying transverse processes, and the lamina at the spinolaminar junction. On the axial CT image at C6 can be seen an enlarged, deformed transverse process on the right with sclerosis that extends into the vertebral body. The osteoblastoma nidus involves the transverse process. Interestingly, when the nidus of an osteoid osteoma involves the lamina, enlargement of the adjacent transverse process may occur.

Between 25% and 50% of osteoblastomas are found in the spine. The most common locations for spinal osteoblastoma (and the smaller osteoid osteoma) are the transverse processes and posterior elements. Osteoblastoma may have a lucent or ossified center. It is usually differentiated from osteoid osteoma by size, with osteoblastoma being larger than 1.5 to 2 cm. The overall appearance can be that of a densely calcified mass, as here, or an expansile, amorphous mass with margins that are often well defined. Regardless of whether osteoblastoma involves the vertebral body alone (in about 10% of cases) or the posterior elements as well, diffuse sclerosis of the vertebral body may result and produce a radiographic "ivory vertebra." Reactive sclerosis at multiple levels has also been reported. Soft tissue masses and epidural extension, as well as postcontrast enhancement of the tumor, are well shown by CT and MR imaging.

Notes

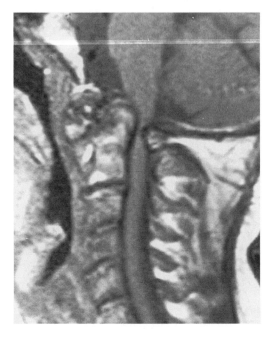
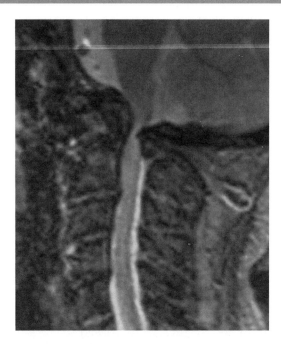

1. Name three congenital disorders associated with an increased prevalence of atlantoaxial dislocation.

2. Name three osseous malformations that may result in atlantoaxial dislocation.

3. Is atlantoaxial subluxation more frequently associated with the adult or the juvenile form of rheumatoid arthritis (RA)?

4. What percentage of children with juvenile rheumatoid arthritis (JRA) test seropositive for rheumatoid factor?

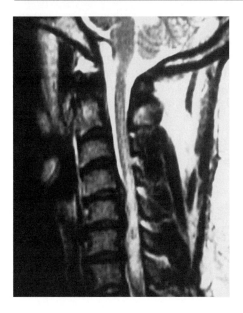
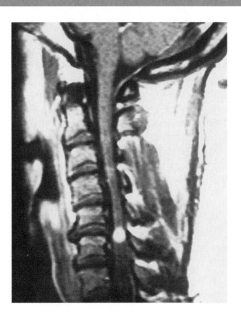
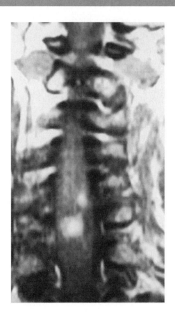

1. This non-AIDS patient has a history of leptomeningeal disease. List three conditions that may cause the findings shown on the T2-weighted and postcontrast T1-weighted images.

2. How might these lesions have arisen?

3. Name at least three intramedullary lesions that occur in patients with AIDS.

4. Which of the lesions listed above may be hypointense or isointense relative to cord on T2-weighted images?

Juvenile Rheumatoid Arthritis

1. Down syndrome, Marfan syndrome, and neurofibromatosis.

2. Os odontoideum, ossiculum terminale, and agenesis of the odontoid base.

3. Adult.

4. 10% to 20%.

Reference

Reiter MF, Boden SD: Inflammatory disorders of the cervical spine. *Spine* 23:2755–2766, 1998.

Cross-Reference

Neuroradiology: THE REQUISITES, p 501.

Comment

The T1- and T2*-weighted sagittal images demonstrate severe compression of the spinal cord near the cervicomedullary junction as a result of atlantoaxial subluxation. The anterior aspect of the dens is irregularly concave. Inhomogeneous signal material representing pannus is interposed between the dens and the anterior arch of C1 (the roughly oval hyperintensity on the T1-weighted image abutting the prevertebral muscles). No abnormal signal intensity is detected within the cord.

JRA is a heterogeneous disease with onset before the age of 16 years (peak at 1 to 3 years); the majority of patients are seronegative for rheumatoid factor. Three distinct clinical manifestations are recognized: polyarticular (50% of patients, resembles adult RA), monoarticular or pauciarticular (30%, best prognosis), and systemic (20%, Still's disease with fever, splenomegaly, lymphadenopathy, rash, pericarditis and myocarditis, and often mild polyarthritis). Spondylitis, which affects the synovium-lined joints of the cervical spine primarily, occurs in 66% of patients with JRA of at least 10 years' duration. Facet (apophyseal) joint changes, especially fusion (increasing from caudad to cephalad), are the most common findings. Subluxation from ligamentous laxity and vertebral body fusion also occur. Atlantoaxial dislocation secondary to destructive granulation tissue (pannus) is relatively uncommon in JRA, compared with adult RA. Patients with JRA who have onset of the disease in very early childhood experience abnormal vertebral development, such as undergrowth of vertebral bodies and intervertebral disks.

Notes

Sarcoidosis, Cervical

1. Metastatic disease, sarcoidosis, and lymphoma.

2. Given the history of leptomeningeal disease, the cord lesions are more likely to be a result of infiltration of the Virchow-Robin spaces than a result of hematogenous spread to the cord.

3. Cytomegalovirus, herpes simplex, and herpes zoster infections, as well as vacuolar myelopathy, tuberculosis, toxoplasmosis, and non-Hodgkin's lymphoma.

4. Lymphomatous, toxoplasmic, and granulomatous (sarcoid, as shown here) lesions.

Reference

Christoforidis GA, Spickler EM, Recio MV, Mehta BM: MR of CNS sarcoidosis: Correlation of imaging features to clinical symptoms and response to treatment. *AJNR Am J Neuroradiol* 20:655–669, 1999.

Cross-Reference

Neuroradiology: THE REQUISITES, p 480.

Comment

The postcontrast T1-weighted coronal image shows two nodular enhancing intramedullary lesions. The larger one, located at C5-6, is evident on the sagittal images and is isointense relative to normal cord on the T2-weighted image. In addition, hyperintense edema is extending from C4 through C7, with cord enlargement at C6-7. Degenerative canal stenosis at C4-5 and C5-6 limits cord expansion. An important clue in this case is the history of leptomeningeal disease, although leptomeningeal enhancement is not convincingly shown on these images. Among patients with sarcoidosis, 5% have clinical neurologic involvement. In autopsy studies, however, 14% to 27% of cases have neurologic involvement pathologically, thus suggesting considerable subclinical disease. The most common clinical symptom of spinal sarcoidosis is weakness. Histopathologically, sarcoid lesions represent a granulomatous meningitis with nodular studding of the cord surface. Infiltration of the perivascular spaces results in the formation of intramedullary granulomas (although pure intramedullary lesions have been described). Although lesions may occur throughout the spinal cord, they are reportedly more frequent in the cervical region. On MR images, the lesions are characterized by (1) cord swelling, (2) increased or mixed (increased and decreased) signal intensity on T2-weighted images, and (3) postcontrast enhancement that is multifocal, patchy or nodular, and located predominantly in the periphery of the cord.

Notes

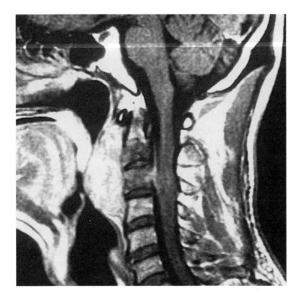
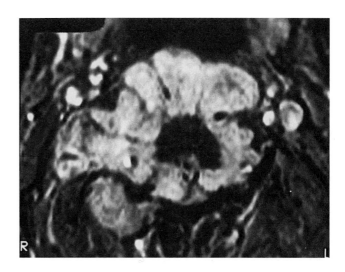

1. What findings on the MR images (postcontrast T1-weighted spin-echo image and T2*-weighted gradient-echo axial image, C3 level) may suggest the diagnosis?

2. In what fascial space is this lesion most likely to be located?

3. Why is this lesion unlikely to be due to nerve sheath tumors?

4. What is ecchordosis physaliphora?

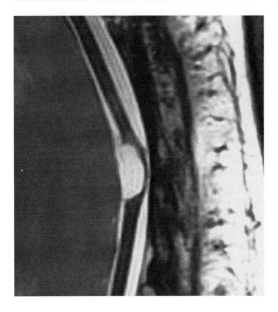
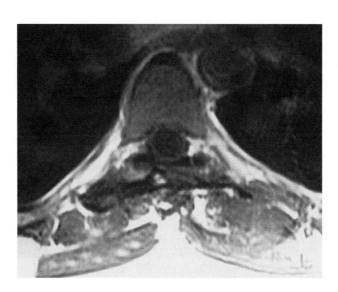

1. Is this T7 lesion, as shown on T2-weighted FSE (fast-spin-echo) sagittal and postcontrast T1-weighted axial images, intramedullary or extramedullary?

2. Is it more likely to be primary (congenital) or secondary (acquired)?

3. Name three congenital intramedullary cystic lesions.

4. What is the frequency of syringomyelia in patients with intradural arachnoid cysts?

Chordoma, Cervical

1. The pattern of hyperintense lobules separated by low-signal intensity septations on the axial image.

2. Prevertebral space.

3. The mass does not follow the course of the spinal nerves on the axial image, and the sagittal image shows evidence of C2 and C3 vertebral involvement.

4. Embryonic ectopic rests of notochordal tissue found adjacent to the pons in about 2% of autopsies and within the retropharyngeal/prevertebral region.

Reference

Wippold FJ 2nd, Koeller KK, Smirniotopoulos JG: Clinical and imaging features of cervical chordoma. *AJR Am J Roentgenol* 172:1423–1426, 1999.

Cross-Reference

Neuroradiology: THE REQUISITES, pp 436, 494.

Comment

The postcontrast T1-weighted image shows a prevertebral mass extending from the atlantooccipital junction to C4, with a tail continuing inferiorly to C5 and epidural/dural enhancement posterior to the C2 and C3 bodies. These vertebral bodies are relatively hypointense in comparison with the remaining cervical vertebrae as a result of tumor-related osteosclerotic and lytic changes of C2 and C3. On the axial gradient-echo image, the perivertebral and bilateral neural foraminal mass is heterogeneously hyperintense and has a lobular contour with hypointense septations separating the lobules. This appearance is characteristic of typical chordomas, in which fibrous strands (accounting for the hypointense septations) create lobules of either mucin-containing physaliphorous cells or purely cystic mucinous pools (accounting for the hyperintensity). The mass is primarily perivertebral, which may be the result of tumor extension from the most frequent site of involvement, the vertebral body, or may represent growth originating from one of the extraosseous notochordal rests (ecchordoses) known to exist in this region. The bilateral neural foraminal (epidural) portion of the tumor protrudes into the canal and is compressing the cord from both sides, which causes a triangle-shaped cord (slightly hypointense to tumor) on the axial image and an apparent focal enlargement of the cord on the sagittal image.

Cervical chordomas usually span several vertebral segments and spare the posterior elements. CT is useful for detecting calcifications and osteosclerosis. Lesions typically included in the differential diagnosis are metastasis, lymphoma, nerve sheath tumor, and osteomyelitis.

Notes

Arachnoid Cyst (Postsurgical), Thoracic

1. The lesion was found to be extramedullary at surgery.

2. Secondary.

3. Hydromyelia, ependymal cyst, and epidermoid.

4. In one study of surgically proven congenital intradural arachnoid cysts, 1 patient in 17 (about 6%) had syringomyelia. For secondary arachnoid cysts, the frequency is probably higher.

Reference

Silbergleit R, Brunberg JA, Patel SC, Mehta BA, Aravapalli SR: Imaging of spinal intradural arachnoid cysts: MRI, myelography, and CT. *Neuroradiology* 40:664–668, 1998.

Cross-Reference

Neuroradiology: THE REQUISITES, p 484.

Comment

The T7 cystic mass deforming the cord has signal characteristics of CSF. Although the margins formed by the anteriorly located cyst and the cord approach 90°, they are slightly obtuse, with evidence of multiple laminectomies. Thus, an acquired intradural extramedullary arachnoid cyst should be favored in the differential diagnosis, which also includes neuroepithelial, enterogenous (neurenteric), and infectious (parasitic) cysts. An enterogenous cyst, which is associated with vertebral body developmental defects, is less likely because of the absence of such defects in this case and because of the relative rarity of this lesion. A neurenteric cyst may be indistinguishable from an arachnoid cyst on MR imaging. Primary arachnoid cysts are usually posterior to the cord and may be related to the septum posticum in the midthoracic region. Arachnoid cysts that occur secondary to trauma, previous surgery, subarachnoid hemorrhage, or infection have been called subarachnoid cysts, but differentiation between primary and secondary cysts may be difficult, so both are often called simply arachnoid cysts. Subarachnoid cysts are occasionally associated with syringomyelia.

In the classification of dural and arachnoid meningeal cysts proposed by Nabors and colleagues, *intradural* arachnoid cysts are called type III spinal meningeal cysts. These defects differ from *extradural* meningeal cysts with (type I) or without (type II) spinal nerve root fibers. Intradural, extramedullary arachnoid cysts may communicate with the subarachnoid space via a wide or narrow neck, presumably affecting their rate of opacification with intrathecal iodinated contrast material, or they may be isolated from the subarachnoid space.

Notes

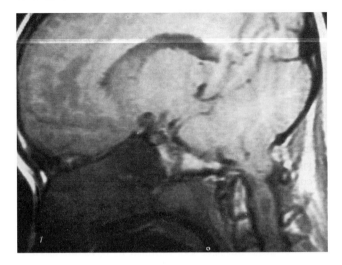

1. Which craniometric measurement is abnormal on this image: Welcker's basal angle, the clivus-canal angle, and/or the atlantooccipital joint axis angle?

2. What associations exist between the craniometric abnormality and the spinal cord findings?

3. In patients with the Chiari I malformation, what is the prevalence of syringohydromyelia?

4. Is basilar invagination present?

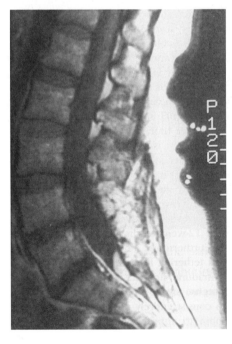
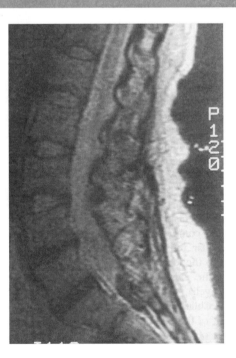

1. Give a differential diagnosis for the intradural mass shown on the T1- and T2-weighted images.

2. Which study would best differentiate these lesions—short tau inversion recovery (STIR) MR imaging or CT scan?

3. What additional findings on MR imaging provide clues to the origin of the mass?

4. List three factors that may contribute to the low-intensity CSF signal in the lumbar subarachnoid space relative to the thoracic subarachnoid space on the T2-weighted image.

Vascular Malformation

1. Supine.

2. Spinal cord, cauda equina, and intradural vessels.

3. Intradural veins located on the surface of the cord.

4. Gadolinium-enhanced MR angiography of the spine.

References

Bowen BC, DePrima S, Pattany PM, Marcillo A, Madsen P, Quencer RM: MR angiography of normal intradural vessels of the thoracolumbar spine. *AJNR Am J Neuroradiol* 17:483-494, 1996.

Thron AK: *Vascular Anatomy of the Spinal Cord.* New York, Springer-Verlag, 1988, pp 65-66.

Cross-Reference

Neuroradiology: THE REQUISITES, pp 496-498.

Comment

The anteroposterior view from a myelogram of the lower thoracic spine shows serpentine filling defects that extend over several vertebral levels, with a "nidus" at the upper intervertebral disk space. These defects are vessels—specifically, enlarged veins on the surface of the cord that are draining blood from an intramedullary or perimedullary arteriovenous malformation (AVM). These veins are part of the coronal venous plexus, a network of vessels encompassing the surface of the cord and containing dominant channels with a cephalocaudad orientation. Abnormal veins are distinguished qualitatively from normal ones only by the greater tortuosity, size, and number of visible vessels; hence, normal and abnormal veins may have similar appearances. For most dural fistulas and intramedullary AVMs, the abnormal veins are most prominent on the posterior surface of the cord. Thus, radiographs obtained during myelography are done with the patient supine. Medullary (or radiculomedullary) veins, which extend from the cord surface to the dura near a neural foramen and drain blood from the cord, may also be detected. Display of normal and abnormal intradural vessels, however, may be obtained directly and more easily by gadolinium-enhanced MR angiography, which has therefore become preferable to supine myelography as a screening technique for spinal vascular malformations (especially dural arteriovenous fistulas).

Notes

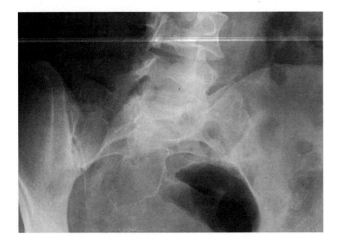
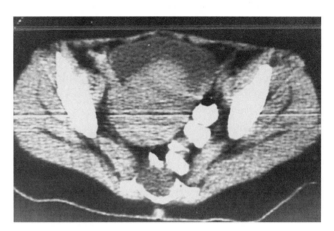

1. What is a "scimitar sacrum"?

2. This appearance is associated with a lesion found in certain congenital disorders or syndromes; name the lesion and two such disorders.

3. Name three primary neoplasms of the sacrum that can produce the findings shown on the plain radiograph and CT scan.

4. As a next step, would you obtain a CT myelogram or an MR scan?

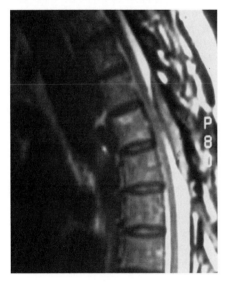
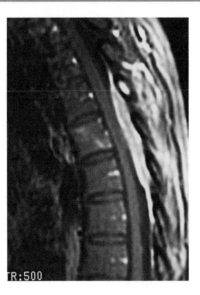

1. The abnormalities shown on the FSE (fast-spin-echo) T2-weighted image and on the postcontrast T1-weighted image involve which spinal space or spaces?

2. What additional image is crucial to narrowing the differential diagnosis, and why?

3. What finding on the T2-weighted image may help further narrow the differential diagnosis?

4. Is metastasis or hematopoietic malignancy more likely to cause signal changes limited to the vertebral body and pedicles?

Anterior Sacral Meningocele

1. As seen on a frontal radiograph of the pelvis, the sacrum demonstrates a smooth, sharply marginated, curvilinear lucent defect. Typically, the defect is unilateral.

2. The lesion is an anterior sacral meningocele, which has been observed in conditions with dural ectasia, such as neurofibromatosis and Marfan syndrome.

3. Giant cell tumor, chordoma, and plasmacytoma.

4. In cases in which an anterior sacral meningocele is possible, MR imaging is preferable to myelography/CT myelography because the latter tests have a significant false-negative rate from obstruction of the meningocele pedicle.

References

McGuire RA Jr, Metcalf JC, Amundson GM, McGillicudy GT: Anterior sacral meningocele. Case report and review of the literature. *Spine* 15:612–614, 1990.

North RB, Kidd DH, Wang H: Occult, bilateral anterior sacral and intrasacral meningeal and perineurial cysts: Case report and review of the literature. *Neurosurgery* 27:981–986, 1990.

Cross-Reference

Neuroradiology: THE REQUISITES, pp 273–274, 484.

Comment

A lytic lesion with a sharp, sclerotic margin near the midline is shown on the oblique frontal radiograph. The CT scan, obtained without intravenous contrast but with oral contrast administration, demonstrates a hypodense mass eroding the anterior, lower portion of the sacrum. This appearance could be due to a relatively nonaggressive tumor or a meningeal cyst, and MR imaging would be more useful in trying to differentiate these possibilities. Meningeal cysts have been classified into three types based on the morphology, location (extradural types I and II versus intradural type III), and absence (type I) or presence (type II) of nerve roots in the cyst. Type II cysts are dilatations of the spinal nerve root sleeves often found in the sacral region (Tarlov cysts). They may enlarge and cause bone erosion, but usually not to the degree shown here. A special category of type I cyst is the relatively rare anterior sacral meningocele (type Ib). This cyst is a diverticulum of the thecal sac that protrudes into the presacral space, usually through a defect in the anterior surface of the sacrum. It has thin walls composed of an outer layer of dura and an inner arachnoid membrane and typically communicates with the intraspinal thecal sac by a narrow stalk. Most anterior sacral meningoceles are congenital, become evident in the second and third decades, and occur in women. In as many as 20% of cases, nerve roots and the filum or spinal ganglia may be found within the meningocele sac or in the sac wall. In 20% of cases the sacral defect responsible for the "scimitar sacrum" sign is midline.

Notes

Lymphoma

1. Epidural and vertebral.

2. Precontrast T1-weighted image to determine whether the epidural collection or mass is hyperintense, which would be suggestive of subacute hematoma. The epidural mass proved to be isointense relative to cord.

3. The relatively low signal intensity in about half the epidural mass on the T2-weighted image.

4. Metastasis.

References

Kim JK, Ryu KN, Choi WS, Choe BK, Choi JM, Yoon AY: Spinal involvement of hematopoietic malignancies and metastasis: Differentiation using MR imaging. *Clin Imaging* 23:125–133, 1999.

Mascalchi M, Torselli P, Falaschi F, Dal Pozzo G: MRI of spinal epidural lymphoma. *Neuroradiology* 37:303–307, 1995.

Cross-Reference

Neuroradiology: THE REQUISITES, p 491.

Comment

The T2-weighted image shows a posteriorly located mass in the upper thoracic canal. The loss of epidural fat signal, which is present more inferiorly, and compression of the subarachnoid space indicate an epidural mass. If the mass is isointense relative to cord on the precontrast T1-weighted image, one may conclude that the postcontrast image demonstrates homogeneous enhancement, and the differential diagnosis includes metastasis, leukemia, lymphoma, myeloma, sarcoma, and possibly meningioma, abscess, or organized hematoma. The differential may be narrowed by three observations: the mass is isointense relative to cord on the T2-weighted images (except for some partial volume averaging with CSF in the lower half of the mass), the vertebral bodies are diffusely hypointense on the postcontrast T1-weighted image (except for the enhancing vertebral body, which is anterior to the epidural mass), and the posterior vertebral elements at the upper extent of the epidural mass are involved. The combination of infiltrative epidural growth (four vertebral levels with minimal cord compression), low signal intensity on T2-weighted images, homogeneous enhancement, and diffuse vertebral marrow signal changes strongly favors lymphoma.

Notes

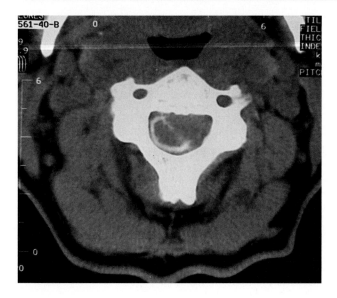

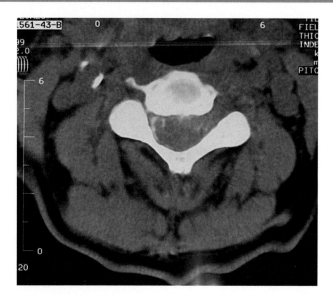

1. Based on these axial CT images at C3 and C3-4, what is the location of the lesion?

2. Name an extramedullary intradural lesion that may be more easily diagnosed with CT myelography than with MR imaging.

3. For extradural meningiomas, is the frequency of hyperostosis in spinal tumors higher than, lower than, or equal to that in cranial tumors?

4. What is the ratio of intradural to extradural spinal meningiomas?

Meningioma, Cervical

1. The mass is extradural in location at C3; however, at C3-4, intrinsic irregularity of the intrathecal contrast suggests an intradural component.

2. Arachnoid cyst.

3. Lower.

4. Approximately 20:1.

Reference

Weil SM, Gewirtz RJ, Tew JM Jr: Concurrent intradural and extradural meningiomas of the cervical spine. *Neurosurgery* 27:629–631, 1990.

Cross-Reference

Neuroradiology: THE REQUISITES, p 489.

Comment

CT myelography was performed on a 71-year-old woman with a history of progressive myeloradiculopathy and burning dysesthetic pain. The axial image at the level of the pedicles of C3 shows contrast in the thecal sac, which is compressed by an extradural mass. At the level of the C3-4 neural foramina, however, the sac is irregularly and asymmetrically filled with contrast— more consistent with an intradural than an extradural location for the mass. At surgery, meningioma with both intradural and extradural components was found. Although myelography and postmyelography CT may be used to identify intradural or extradural masses, these techniques are often confined to merely establishing the presence of a "block" and its level. If contrast was instilled through a lumbar puncture, a C1-2 puncture might be required to delineate the spinal canal cephalic to the level of a complete "block." For this and other reasons, MR imaging is preferred for evaluation of myelopathy.

The most frequent location for intraspinal meningiomas is the thoracic spine (about 80%), followed by the cervical spine. Most of these tumors are intradural, with less than 15% being extradural or combined intradural and extradural. In many of the reported cases of purely extradural meningioma, the lesions had not been explored intradurally, so combined lesions may be more common than was previously estimated. Concurrent meningiomas may also occur and should thus prompt evaluation of both the intradural space and extradural space for lesions. In one report, two meningiomas, an extradural fibrous meningioma and an intradural syncytial meningioma, not in continuity, were found at the same spinal level (C2-3).

Notes

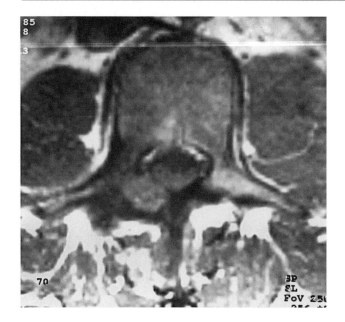

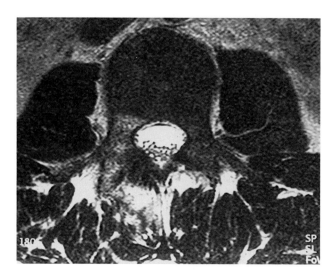

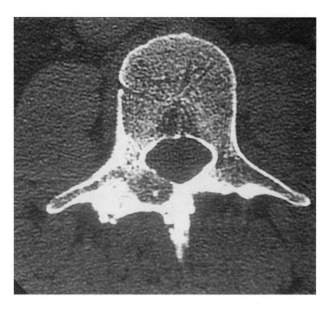

1. What is the differential diagnosis for a dense pedicle seen on plain radiographs?

2. How do you explain the sclerotic thickening of the right transverse process of L3 in this case?

3. Where is the lesion located? Is this site atypical?

4. Do you expect this 28-year-old man to have local or radicular pain?

Osteoid Osteoma, Lumbar

1. Osteoblastic metastasis, enostosis (bone island), osteoid osteoma (or the larger osteoblastoma), atypical infection, lymphoma, and reactive sclerosis secondary to abnormal facets (congenital or degenerative).

2. As a reaction to the laminar osteoid osteoma.

3. Right lamina. No. In osteoid osteoma, the laminae are the most commonly affected parts of the vertebra. With metastasis, the pedicles are more commonly affected than the laminae or other posterior elements.

4. Patients almost always have local pain. Radicular pain, presumably arising from encroachment of the lesion on the neural foramen, occurs in about 50% of patients.

Reference

Murphey MD, Andrews CL, Flemming DJ, Temple HT, Smith WS, Smirniotopoulos JG: From the archives of the AFIP. Primary tumors of the spine: Radiologic pathologic correlation. *Radiographics* 16:1131–1158, 1996.

Cross-Reference

Neuroradiology: THE REQUISITES, p 494.

Comment

CT is the study of choice in the evaluation of suspected osteoid osteoma. The classic finding, as shown here, is a small (<1.5 cm) rounded area of low attenuation, with or without central calcification, surrounded by a variable zone of sclerosis. The lesion is located in the right lamina, and sclerotic changes are evident in the pedicle and transverse process. The right lamina and transverse process are thickened. MR findings are less characteristic. On the T1-weighted image, the nidus is approximately isointense relative to the vertebral body and hyperintense relative to the contralateral lamina. Postcontrast images (not shown) demonstrate mild enhancement, although striking enhancement has been described in the literature as a feature of the vascular nidus. Hypointensity of the right pedicle probably reflects the sclerosis seen on the CT image, as well as edema/inflammation. The latter is inferred from the hyperintensity of the pedicle on the T2-weighted fast-spin-echo image. Interestingly, the nidus in this case is isointense relative to the surrounding sclerotic posterior elements and to the vertebral body, rather than hyperintense, as has been reported for the noncalcified portion of the nidus on long recovery time (TR) standard spin-echo images. Hyperintensity in the adjacent retrospinal soft tissues reportedly represents reactive inflammation.

About 10% of cases of osteoid osteoma involve the axial skeleton. The pain associated with the lesion is classically nocturnal and is relieved by salicylates or nonsteroidal antiinflammatory medication. Affected patients are usually 10 to 20 years of age and are predominantly male (2:1 to 3:1). Clinically, "painful scoliosis" may be a clue to the diagnosis. The posterior elements are involved in 75% of cases and the vertebral body is involved in only 7%. The lesion is located in the lamina in 33% of cases, the articular facets in 19%, and the pedicles in 15%. The nidus consists of vascular connective tissue with surrounding osteoid matrix. The extent of the sclerotic bony reaction around the nidus is variable and may include the entire vertebral body as well as the adjacent vertebrae. In the spine, the lumbar region is most commonly affected (59% of cases).

Notes

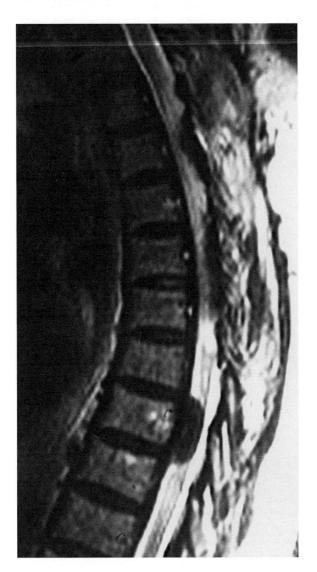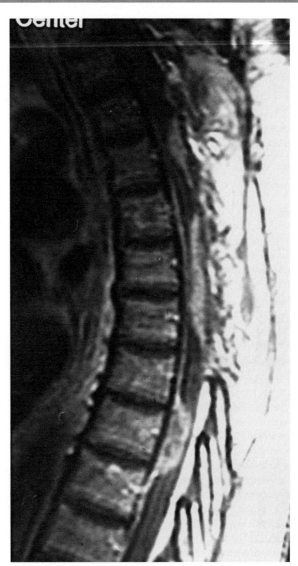

1. Are the lesions shown on the T2-weighted and postcontrast T1-weighted images likely to be extradural, intradural extramedullary, and/or intramedullary in location?

2. How would you account for the multiple sites?

3. Name three primary CNS tumors that metastasize to sites outside the CNS.

4. Are the lesions shown here more likely to be benign or malignant?

C A S E   1 0 9

Multiple Meningiomas, Thoracic

1. Intradural extramedullary (inferiorly) and extradural (superiorly).

2. Either spread through the subarachnoid space or a clustering phenomenon of meningotheliomatous cell aggregates.

3. Meningioma, primitive neuroectodermal tumor (medulloblastoma), and glioblastoma multiforme.

4. Benign.

References

Butti G, Assietti R, Casalone R, Paoletti P: Multiple meningiomas: A clinical, surgical, and cytogenetic analysis. *Surg Neurol* 31:255-260, 1989.

Lee TT, Landy HJ: Spinal metastases of malignant intracranial meningioma. *Surg Neurol* 50:437-441, 1998.

Cross-Reference

Neuroradiology: THE REQUISITES, p 489.

Comment

Evidence of previous multilevel laminectomy is apparent, and three markedly hypointense masses protrude into the upper thoracic canal on the T2-weighted image. The cord is compressed and has increased signal intensity in the same region. Each of the masses exhibits prominent enhancement with intravenous gadolinium. The most inferiorly located mass (T7 level) produces widening of the subarachnoid space anterior to the cord, consistent with an intradural extramedullary location. On the postcontrast T1-weighted image, this mass demonstrates inhomogeneous enhancement with a "dural tail" sign. This sign, which reportedly occurs in up to 70% of intracranial meningiomas, is less commonly associated with dural metastases and is rarely observed in association with nerve sheath tumors. Because of the previous surgery, it is difficult to determine whether the remaining, homogeneously enhancing lesions (T1 through T5 levels) have both extradural and intradural components.

Some investigators use the term "multiple meningiomas" to refer to a condition in which at least two tumors are present at different sites in patients without signs of neurofibromatosis, regardless of the chronology of appearance of the tumors. Based on several autopsy studies, the frequency of occurrence of multiple meningiomas is believed to be about 8% to 10%. One hypothesis regarding the pathogenesis of multiple meningiomas is that in each case they originated from one tumor that has undergone desquamation and spread through the subarachnoid space to other sites. This hypothesis has been challenged on the basis that the karyotype differs from tumor to tumor in the same patient. In addition, it has been shown that the dura in the region of a single meningioma contains many clusters of meningotheliomatous cell ("cap" cell) aggregates. Because meningiomas are thought to arise from "cap" cells, this regional multicentricity has been proposed as an alternative hypothesis to explain the existence of nearby meningiomas, whether intradural, extradural, or both.

Malignant intracranial meningioma metastasizing to the spinal subarachnoid space/nerve roots is rare, with fewer than 20 reported cases. Patients with such metastases tend to be male and to have undergone multiple resections of intracranial lesions. Recently reported cases with contrast-enhanced MR imaging show nodular enhancing lesions along the conus medullaris and roots of the cauda equina. Extracranial metastases to the lung, lymph nodes, and abdominal organs have also been reported.

Notes

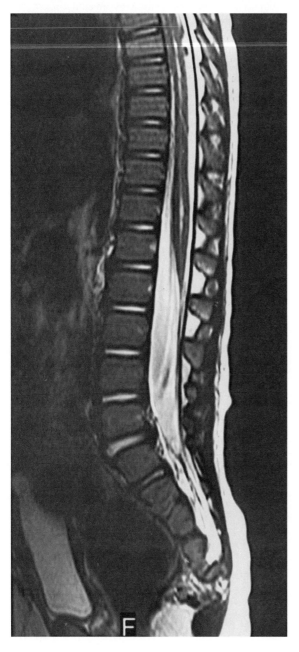

1. In this 3-year-old boy with a history of imperforate anus, what findings should be searched for on this sagittal T2-weighted fast-spin-echo image?

2. Which two embryologic processes are responsible for formation of the ventriculus terminalis, or "fifth ventricle"?

3. Which of these two is probably anomalous in this case?

4. Give at least four examples of occult spinal dysraphism.

Terminal Ventricle and Hydromyelia

1. Cord tethering and/or a presacral mass.

2. (1) Neurulation and (2) canalization and retrogressive differentiation.

3. Canalization and retrogressive differentiation of the "caudal cell mass."

4. Diastematomyelia, lipomyelomeningocele, meningocele manqué, dermal sinus tract (with dermoid cyst), neurenteric cyst, and tight filum terminale (with tethered cord).

References

Coleman LT, Zimmerman RA, Rorke LB: Ventriculus terminalis of the conus medullaris: MR findings in children. *AJNR Am J Neuroradiol* 16:1421-1426, 1995.

Gegg CA, Vollmer DG, Tullous MW, Kagan-Hallet KS: An unusual case of the complete Currarino triad: Case report, discussion of the literature and the embryogenic implications. *Neurosurgery* 44:658-62, 1999.

Iskandar BJ, Oakes WJ, McLaughlin C, Osumi AK, Tien RD: Terminal syringohydromyelia and occult spinal dysraphism. *J Neurosurg* 81:513-519, 1994.

Cross-Reference

Neuroradiology: THE REQUISITES, pp 274-276.

Comment

The midsagittal image shows some deformity of the sacrococcygeal junction, a normally positioned conus with its tip at L2, and a narrow, centrally located, intramedullary cystic region from T6 through L1. In an asymptomatic child, the cystic region may be viewed as an incidental finding and described as a ventriculus terminalis (terminal ventricle) and/or idiopathic localized hydromyelia. Although small in diameter, the cystic region involves approximately the caudal third of the cord, and in a child with imperforate anus, the possibility of hydromyelia (or more generally, syringohydromyelia) should be considered. "Terminal syringohydromyelia" is defined by Iskandar and associates as an intramedullary cyst located in the caudal third of the cord that when large is often symptomatic and requires treatment. In one study of 143 cases of occult spinal dysraphism, 24 terminal syringes were identified by MR imaging. Ten of the syringes were small; however, their appearance was described as spherical (<2 cm in diameter) rather than elongated, as in this case. An important consideration for this case was that among the 24 patients with terminal syringes, a relatively high incidence (67%) of terminal syringohydromyelia was noted in the tethered cord/anorectal malformation group (6 of 9 cases). Thus, it is important to note the position and contour of the conus tip, as well as the presence of an intramedullary cyst, when reporting the MR imaging findings in a patient with imperforate anus or anorectal stenosis. Fortunately for this patient, no evidence of cord tethering can be seen. Another association pertinent to this case is that of anorectal malformation, anterior sacral defect, and presacral mass (Currarino's triad). Among patients with this triad, the incidence of tethered cord is about 20%.

Anomalies involving the filum and the sacrococcygeal spinal segments, with or without anorectal/urogenital malformations, are thought to be the result of aberrant canalization and retrogressive differentiation of the caudal cell mass, a large aggregate of undifferentiated cells that includes the caudal end of the neural tube and the caudal end of the notochord. The terminal ventricle, which is a normal slight expansion of the central canal in the distal conus and/or proximal filum, is thought to represent the point of union between the portion of the central canal made by neurulation and the portion made by canalization of the caudal cell mass. Usually, the terminal ventricle disappears in the first 6 months or so after birth. In a study by Coleman and colleagues of 418 children (aged 5 days to 20 years; median age, approximately 5 years) without clinical evidence of spinal disease, a terminal ventricle was identified in 2.6%, with mean measurements of 22 × 4.1 × 4.2 mm.

Notes

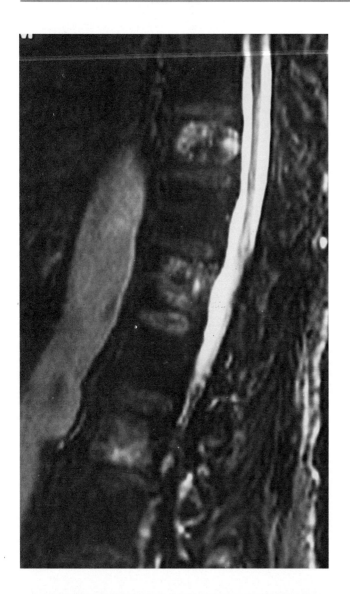

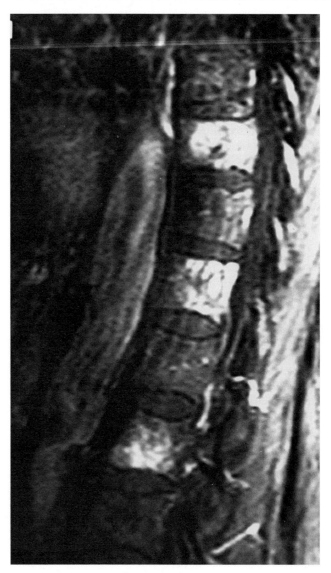

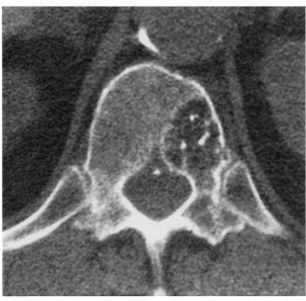

1. List three different types of lesions that can produce the findings shown on the fat-saturated T2-weighted and postcontrast T1-weighted MR images, and demonstrate uptake on ^{99m}Tc-pertechnetate bone scan.

2. T2-weighted MR imaging with fat suppression (using STIR [short tau inversion recovery] or chemical shift fat saturation) is often recommended to improve detection of vertebral metastases. It may be less helpful in detecting metastases from which primary tumors?

3. Do the majority of spinal metastases start in the vertebral body or in the pedicle?

4. In this 75-year-old man with a history of prostate cancer, is MR imaging or CT more convincing for a diagnosis of metastatic disease?

Multiple Vertebral Hemangiomas

1. Metastases, hemangiomas, and lymphoma.

2. Tumors that produce osteoblastic (sclerotic) metastases, such as prostate and carcinoid.

3. Vertebral body and subsequently grow into the region of the pedicle and posterior elements.

4. MR findings for the lesions at T10, T12, and L2 are consistent with metastases, whereas the CT findings (here shown for the T12 lesion) favor hemangioma.

Reference

Kulshrestha M, Byrne P: Multiple primary haemangiomas of bone mimicking vertebral metastases. *J R Soc Med* 90:632–634, 1997.

Cross-Reference

Neuroradiology: THE REQUISITES, pp 493–494.

Comment

On the fat-saturated T2-weighted MR image, increased signal intensity is seen within the T10, T12, and L2 vertebral bodies from end-plate to end-plate, with a mottled appearance. The lesions show marked enhancement, yet no loss of vertebral body height and no epidural extension are apparent. The multifocal findings are clearly consistent with but not limited to metastatic disease. Both bone scan and CT were recommended for this patient. The bone scan demonstrated uptake in the vertebral bodies in question, as well as in a rib, again suggesting metastatic disease. CT, however, showed lesions with low-density (less than −30 HU) stroma within an osseous network, thickening of some of the bony "trabeculae," and an intact vertebral cortex. A diagnosis of multiple hemangiomas was confirmed by comparison with a plain radiograph that had been obtained years earlier.

Hemangiomas are routinely hyperintense on T2-weighted images, as seen for the lesions in this case. The hyperintensity has been attributed to increased water content, presumably associated with the angiomatous component of the stroma, which coexists with the fatty component. On postcontrast, fat-saturated T1-weighted images, the degree of enhancement reflects the extent of vascularization of the stroma and ranges from intense enhancement in aggressive (often symptomatic) hemangiomas to minimal or no enhancement in indolent (asymptomatic) hemangiomas. The MR image features of hemangiomas overlap with those of metastases from prostate, breast, lung, and renal cell carcinomas. Many but by no means all prostate metastases appear sclerotic on plain radiographs and hypointense on both T1- and T2-weighted images, thus distinguishing them from the hemangiomas shown here. Schmorl (cited in the reference above) found hemangiomas of the vertebral body in almost 11% of necropsies. The most common sites, in order of frequency, were T12, L4, L1, L2, and L3.

Notes

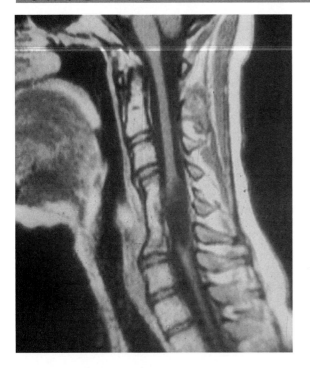

1. What surgical procedure has been performed in this patient with a history of cervical trauma?
2. Excluding syringomyelia, list three causes of posttraumatic myelopathy.
3. Which of these causes may be contributing to this patient's myelopathy?
4. What MR pulse sequence may help distinguish a confluent cord cyst from myelomalacia?

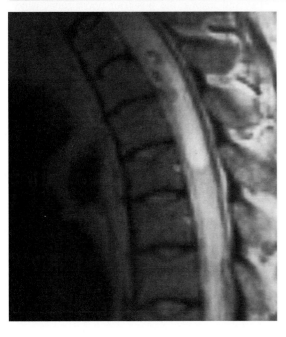
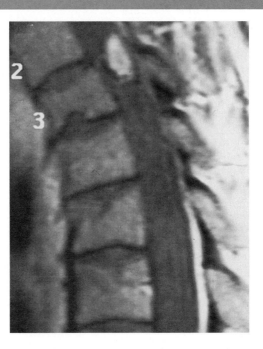

1. Give a differential diagnosis for the findings on the T2-weighted and postcontrast T1-weighted images above.
2. What additional MR imaging would help narrow the differential diagnosis?
3. What is the likelihood that this patient has von Hippel-Lindau disease? In what percentage of patients with von Hippel-Lindau disease does spinal hemangioblastoma develop?
4. Is this patient likely to have erythrocytosis?

Progressive Posttraumatic Myelomalacic Myelopathy*

1. C4 through C6 anterior corpectomy, diskectomy, and fusion.

2. Cord compression by a bone fragment or subarachnoid cyst, cord tethering, and microcystic spinal cord degeneration/gliosis.

3. Cord tethering and microcystic degeneration.

4. Long recovery time (TR)/short echo time (TE) (proton-density-weighted [PDW]) spin-echo sequence. On a PDW image, myelomalacia is typically hyperintense, whereas a cord cyst with signal characteristics of CSF is hypointense relative to uninvolved cord parenchyma.

References

Falcone S, Quencer RM, Green BA, Patchen SJ, Post MJ: Progressive posttraumatic myelomalacic myelopathy: Imaging and clinical features. *AJNR Am J Neuroradiol* 15:747–754, 1994.

Lee TT, Arias JM, Andrus HL, Quencer RM, Falcone SF, Green BA: Progressive posttraumatic myelomalacic myelopathy: Treatment with untethering and expansive duraplasty. *J Neurosurg* 86:624–628, 1997.

Cross-Reference

Neuroradiology: THE REQUISITES, pp 484–485.

Comment

The sagittal T1-weighted image demonstrates focal cord expansion from C4 through C6, posterior to the surgical interbody fusion. The expanded region has irregular margins and signal intensity slightly greater than that of CSF. This finding could be interpreted as a posttraumatic intramedullary cyst or as myelomalacia with cord tethering. T2-weighted images are less likely to resolve the uncertainty than are PDW images, which often show myelomalacia as hyperintense and show confluent cyst as hypointense (CSF equivalent) relative to normal cord. The two lesions may produce similar clinical findings, namely, evidence of progressive myelopathy. Differentiation by MR imaging is valuable because surgical treatment differs for the two lesions: the cord cyst is treated by shunting, whereas myelomalacia with cord tethering appears to benefit from lysis of adhesions and placement of a dural allograft. Differentiation by CT myelography is hampered by the observation (from several investigators) that intrathecal contrast may permeate the myelomalacic cord on delayed (4 hours) CT scans and thus mimic contrast filling of an intramedullary cyst.

The clinical syndrome of progressive myelopathy in patients who have no confluent shuntable intramedullary cyst has been referred to as "progressive posttraumatic myelomalacic myelopathy." Preliminary histopathologic studies of the myelomalacic region have shown reactive astrocytosis, microcysts, and thickening of the pia-arachnoid. Several authors have hypothesized that the microcysts can eventually coalesce to form a confluent cyst (macrocyst).

---

*Figure for Case 112 from Falcone S, Quencer RM, Green BA, Patchen SJ, Post MJ: Progressive posttraumatic myelomalacic myelopathy: Imaging and clinical features. *AJNR Am J Neuroradiol* 15:747–754, 1994.

Hemangioblastoma

1. Hemangioblastoma, arteriovenous malformation, ependymoma, and metastasis.

2. Axial two-dimensional flow-sensitive gradient-echo images or postcontrast three-dimensional MR angiography.

3. Approximately 33% of patients with spinal hemangioblastoma have von Hippel-Lindau disease. For patients with the disease, 13% to 59% (the lower percentage is more likely correct) have spinal hemangioblastoma.

4. No. Erythrocytosis occurs when cerebellar hemangioblastoma is present, but it has not been reported to occur with spinal hemangioblastoma.

References

Bowen BC, Latchaw RE: MR angiography of the spinal cord. In: Alexander E III, Maciunas RJ, Eds: *Advanced Neurosurgical Navigation*. New York, Thieme, 1997, pp 49–69.

Choyke PL, Glenn GM, McClellan MW, Patronas NJ, Linehan WM, Zebar B: von Hippel-Lindau disease: Genetic, clinical, and imaging features. *Radiology* 194:629–642, 1995.

Cross-Reference

Neuroradiology: THE REQUISITES, p 487.

Comment

Spinal hemangioblastoma is usually intramedullary and generally involves the thoracic (61%) or cervical (29%) cord, yet it may have an exophytic component. It can be exclusively extramedullary and involve the posterior nerve roots, cauda equina, or filum terminale, and among all tumors involving these sites, hemangioblastoma has an incidence of 4% to 5%. An intramedullary hemangioblastoma is primarily located in the posterior half of the spinal cord and is supplied by the posterior spinal artery or arteries. The tumor consists of a hypervascular nodular mass, usually with an associated cyst (75% of cases) that may contain hemorrhagic components, and a variable degree of surrounding edema. No individual vessels are recognized within the mass angiographically, and arteriovenous shunting is absent. On MR imaging, diffuse cord enlargement often extends over several segments with inhomogeneous signal intensity on T1- and T2-weighted images. Foci of low signal intensity within the cord or on its surface can be due to flowing blood or the magnetic susceptibility effect of hemosiderin. Postcontrast MR angiography is useful to establish these "signal voids" as blood flow within normal-sized or enlarged vessels and to show that some of the vessels are contiguous with the enhancing tumor nodule. The tumor nodule (located here at T2-3) enhances on postcontrast T1-weighted images, whereas the cyst wall and edematous cord do not enhance.

Notes

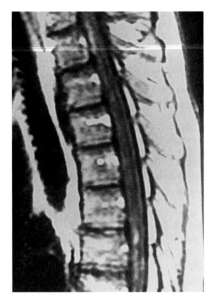
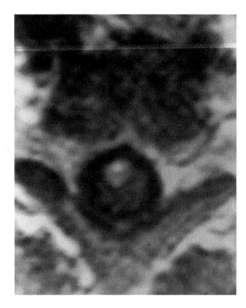

1. Based on the postcontrast T1-weighted sagittal image and the axial image at the C7 level, name three possible causes for myelopathy in this patient with AIDS.

2. Which of these causes can be associated with meningeal as well as cord enhancement?

3. In AIDS patients, what is the frequency of *Toxoplasma* myelitis relative to *Toxoplasma* encephalitis?

4. What is the most common opportunistic infection of the spinal cord in adult AIDS patients?

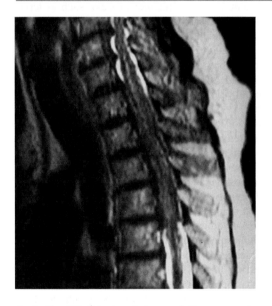
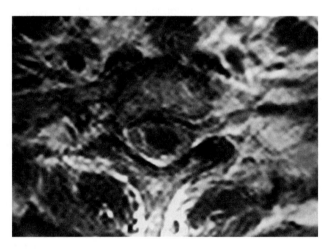

1. Is the T1-4 lesion intramedullary or extramedullary in location?

2. List four common MR imaging features of intramedullary neoplasms.

3. Which features are present on the T2-weighted and postcontrast T1-weighted images?

4. Is cytologic study of CSF obtained by lumbar puncture likely to be positive or negative?

Ependymoma of the Filum Terminale/ Cauda Equina

1. Ependymoma.

2. No.

3. MR imaging of the head and remainder of the spine because of the possibility of subarachnoid dissemination of ependymoma, metastases, or lymphoma.

4. Myxopapillary ependymoma, schwannoma, and dermoid.

Reference

Wippold FJ II, Smirniotopoulos JG, Moran CJ, Suojanen JN, Vollmer DG: MR imaging of myxopapillary ependymoma: Findings and value to determine extent of tumor and its relation to intraspinal structures. *AJR Am J Roentgenol* 165:1263–1267, 1995.

Cross-Reference

Neuroradiology: THE REQUISITES, pp 486–487.

Comment

The precontrast sagittal and postcontrast axial T1-weighted images demonstrate mass-like thickening (isointense to cord) and enhancement in the region of the filum/cauda equina. The differential diagnosis includes intradural extramedullary neoplasms (ependymoma, schwannoma/neurofibroma, meningioma, metastasis, lymphoma, paraganglioma) and infectious/ inflammatory thickening and clumping of the nerve roots (arachnoiditis).

Ependymomas account for 90% of primary tumors in the filum terminale. Spinal ependymomas rarely calcify. In the region of the filum and conus medullaris, 30% to 80% of ependymomas are of the myxopapillary subtype. These highly vascular tumors demonstrate mucinous changes not present in other histologic subtypes of ependymomas. The prominent vascularity accounts in part for the marked enhancement sometimes observed on postcontrast MR images. The subarachnoid hemorrhage that occurs with this tumor can lead to superficial siderosis, which is best shown on T2- or T2*-weighted images. MR imaging findings in myxopapillary ependymomas are nonspecific: hyperintense signal relative to spinal cord on T2-weighted images, isointense to hyperintense signal on T1-weighted images, and homogeneous or heterogeneous enhancement. Some authors have reported an increased frequency of hyperintense myxopapillary lesions on precontrast T1-weighted images when compared with other histologic subtypes and have attributed the difference to the mucinous changes noted above. Subependymoma of the filum has similar signal characteristics but may lack enhancement.

Myxopapillary ependymomas are slow growing, with the typical tumor spanning four vertebral levels. Larger tumors often fill the spinal canal and cause scalloping of the posterior margins of the vertebral bodies. Rare extradural sacral and presacral myxopapillary tumors arise from embryonic ependymal rests, and these masses behave more aggressively. Examples of pulmonary, osseous, and lymph node metastases from these lesions have been reported. When large, they cause sacral destruction and can be confused with chordoma, giant cell tumor, aneurysmal bone cyst, or osseous metastases.

Notes

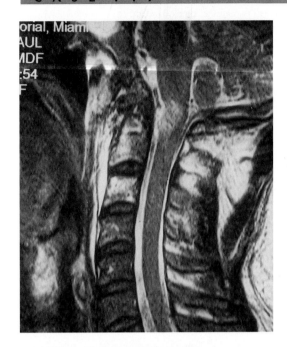
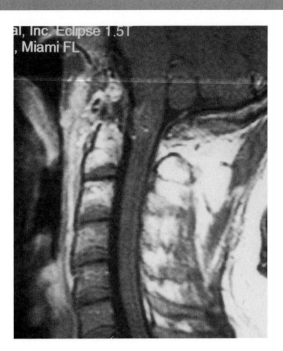
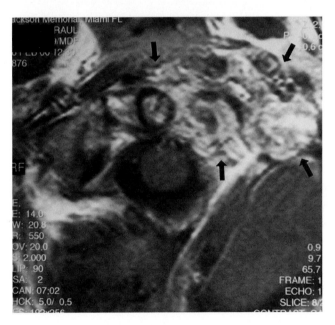

1. Where is this lesion located?

2. How would this lesion be categorized in the classification system of Spetzler and colleagues?

3. What is a metamere, and how is it related to Cobb's syndrome?

4. How are lesions of this type usually treated?

Arteriovenous Malformation (Juvenile Type at C1–C2)

1. Intramedullary, intradural extramedullary, extradural, and extraspinal spaces at C1–C2.

2. Type III (juvenile) arteriovenous malformation (AVM).

3. A metamere is a homologous spinal segment plus neighboring tissue (in the same segmental dermatome) supplied by the corresponding pair of segmental arteries. A metamere includes the cord (myelomeric component), nerve roots, vertebra, paravertebral musculature, subcutaneous tissue, and skin. Cobb's syndrome refers to a metameric vascular malformation involving the triad of skin, bone, and spinal cord. It thus involves structures derived from two or more embryonic layers and represents a "cutaneous vertebral medullary angiomatosis."

4. Staged embolization and, when possible, partial resection.

References

Detweiler PW, Porter RW, Spetzler RF: Spinal arteriovenous malformations. *Neurosurg Clin N Am* 10:89-100, 1999.

Rosenblum B, Oldfield EH, Doppman JL, Di Chiro G: Spinal arteriovenous malformations: A comparison of dural arteriovenous fistulas and intradural AVM's in 81 patients. *J Neurosurg* 67:795-802, 1987.

Cross-Reference

Neuroradiology: THE REQUISITES, pp 496-498.

Comment

At the cervicomedullary junction is an area of patchy, inhomogeneous, increased signal intensity within the cord on the T2-weighted image and linear plus punctate enhancement on the postcontrast T1-weighted images. The enhancing structures are vessels, and they are also seen in the extramedullary intradural space anterolateral to the cord, which is not enlarged. In addition, striking extradural, vertebral, and paraspinal enhancement can be seen anteriorly and to the patient's left at C1–C2 *(arrows)*. The cord findings are consistent with an intramedullary component of the AVM.

Spetzler and colleagues have proposed the following classification system for spinal vascular malformations: type I, dural arteriovenous fistula; type II, intramedullary glomus AVM; type III, intramedullary juvenile AVM; and type IV, intradural (perimedullary) arteriovenous fistula. When compared with a type II glomus AVM with its compact, strictly intramedullary nidus, of a type III juvenile AVM is more diffuse and can involve extramedullary, extradural, and even extraspinal structures (as in this case). Typically, the cervical region is affected. Multiple arterial feeders are present, often from several different vertebral levels. The most common initial symptom in patients with juvenile-type AVM is weakness. This lesion is less prone to hemorrhage than is a glomus-type AVM, which accounts for most cases of symptomatic hemorrhage. Approximately one third of patients with intramedullary AVM have symptoms associated with hemorrhage. Juvenile AVMs occur in adolescents and young adults and have a poor prognosis. The lesions are rarely amenable to direct surgical excision. Treatment consists of endovascular embolization in a staged fashion, sometimes combined with feeder ligation and/or partial resection.

Metameric vascular malformations, as occur in Cobb's syndrome, are not included in the classification system described above. These lesions may be clinically suspected from the cutaneous vascular malformation.

Notes

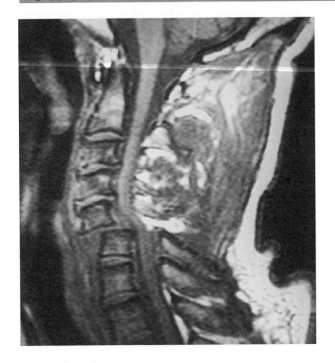

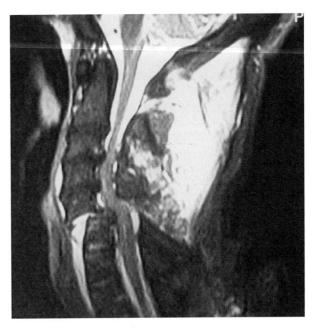

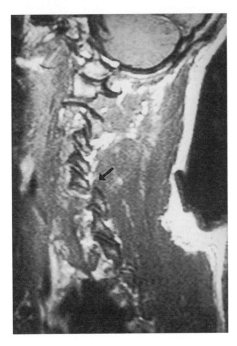

1. Based on the T1-weighted sagittal and right parasagittal images and the T2-weighted image, what is the mechanism of injury? Is the cervical spine likely to be clinically stable or unstable at C5-6, and why?

2. What is the condition of the anterior longitudinal ligament?

3. This 43-year-old man was examined for acute upper extremity weakness, primarily involving the hands, with sparing of the lower extremities and preserved bowel and bladder function. What clinical syndrome does he have?

4. In general, what MR imaging findings in a patient with spine trauma are associated with a poor prognosis?

Bilateral Facet Dislocation With Central Cord Syndrome

1. Flexion-distraction. Unstable, because of disruption of the posterior ligamentous complex, which is inferred from the presence of bilateral facet dislocations and evidence of edema/hemorrhage in the interspinous region above C6.

2. Complete tear, confirmed at surgery.

3. Central cord syndrome.

4. Evidence of intramedullary hemorrhage on T1- and T2-weighted (or T2*-weighted) images. Such evidence is not present in this case.

References

McGuire RA Jr: Physical examination in spinal trauma. In: Levine AM, Eismont FJ, Garfin SR, Zigler JE, Eds: *Spine Trauma*. Philadelphia, WB Saunders, 1998, pp 16-27.

Quencer RM, Bunge RP, Egnor M, et al: Acute traumatic central cord syndrome: MRI-pathological correlations. *Neuroradiology* 34:85-94, 1992.

Cross-Reference

Neuroradiology: THE REQUISITES, pp 498-499.

Comment

This patient was struck on the back of the head by a heavy barrel. The midsagittal T1- and T2-weighted images show anterior displacement of C5 on C6 measuring approximately 60% to 70% of a vertebral body. Bilateral facet injuries are frequently associated with translation greater than 50% of a vertebral body, and in this case the parasagittal images confirmed the presence of bilateral C5-6 facet dislocations (the *arrow* identifies the right facet dislocation). Abnormal signal with increased distance between the C5 and C6 spinous processes indicates interspinous ligament disruption. The heterogeneous signal intensity posterior to the C5 body probably represents epidural blood, as well as a traumatic disk herniation (confirmed at surgery) at C5-6. The spinal cord is compressed, and an associated abnormal intramedullary hyperintensity consistent with edema is present at C6 and C4-5, with no evidence of cord hemorrhage. The anterior longitudinal ligament is disrupted, with edema and/or a fluid collection anterior to C4, C5, and C6 through C7. The patient has osteophytes from C2-3 through C4-5—evidence of underlying chronic degenerative disease.

The central cord syndrome is usually seen in older persons who sustain a cervical hyperextension injury. The spinal cord is injured by a pincer mechanism in which the cord is compressed between vertebral body osteophytes (anterior canal) and hypertrophied/buckled ligamentum flavum (posterior canal). Before 1990, published articles attributed the acute traumatic central cord syndrome (ATCCS) to hemorrhage, necrosis, or contusion within the central portion of the cord, with the more medially coursing fibers (of the upper extremity) affected, as opposed to the more laterally coursing fibers (of the lower extremity) within the lateral corticospinal tracts. This hypothesis was based in part on the results of laboratory studies using animal models. More recent MR imaging-pathologic correlative studies of injured humans have not supported this hypothesis and instead have found the following:

1. MR evidence of hemorrhage is usually absent in cases of ATCCS (as in this case).

2. The central gray matter is intact.

3. Primarily, the spinal cord exhibits diffuse disruption of axons, especially within the lateral columns of the cervical cord in the region occupied by the corticospinal tracts.

Based on these results, Quencer and colleagues have concluded that ATCCS is principally a white matter injury and that the predominant loss of motor function in the distal muscles of the upper limbs reflects the importance of the corticospinal tract for hand and finger function in the primate.

Treatment in this case consisted of reduction of facet dislocation, anterior cervical diskectomy and fusion (C5-6), and subsequent posterior fusion (C5-6). At surgery, tears of the anterior and posterior longitudinal ligaments were found to be complete and almost complete, respectively.

Notes

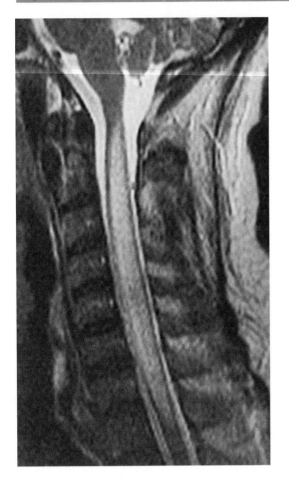

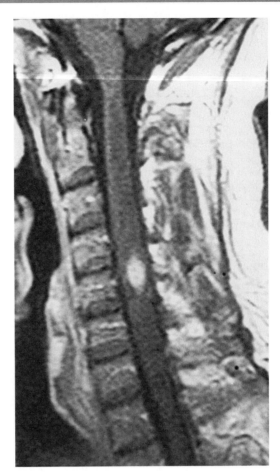

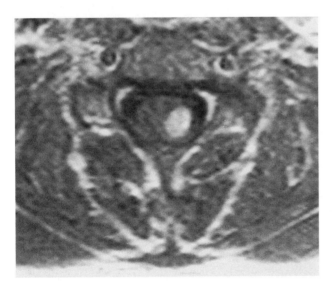

1. List three findings on the T2-weighted and postcontrast T1-weighted images that favor a diagnosis of neoplasm over demyelinating disease.

2. Name three neoplastic lesions that may have this appearance.

3. Why is this lesion unlikely to be an ependymoma?

4. This patient had a negative MR study of the brain. What is the probability that the cervical lesion is a multiple sclerosis (MS) plaque?

Multiple Sclerosis Mimicking Tumor

1. High signal intensity on the T2-weighted image extending over the entire cervical spine and appearing to be centrally located; cord enlargement; and striking nodular enhancement as seen with metastasis.

2. Metastasis (e.g., breast, lung), lymphoma, and hemangioblastoma.

3. An ependymoma of this size is more likely to be centrally located given its origin from ependymal cells of the central canal, and almost 50% of ependymomas have associated cystic cavities (based on autopsy studies).

4. Approximately 10% of patients who meet clinical criteria for MS have lesions identified only in the spinal cord.

References

Lycklama a Nijeholt GJ, Barkhof F, Scheltens P, et al: MR of the spinal cord in multiple sclerosis: Relation to clinical subtype and disability. *AJNR Am J Neuroradiol* 18:1041–1048, 1997.

Tartaglino LM, Friedman DP, Flanders AE, Lublin FD, Knobler RL, Liem M: Multiple sclerosis in the spinal cord: MR appearance and correlation with clinical parameters. *Radiology* 195:725–732, 1995.

Cross-Reference

Neuroradiology: THE REQUISITES, pp 480–481.

Comment

The T2-weighted image shows diffusely increased signal intensity and enlargement of the cervical cord, suggestive of edema. The nodular enhancing lesion at C5 appears to be approximately in the middle of the cord on the sagittal T1-weighted image; however, the axial image demonstrates a left posterolateral cord location.

On T2-weighted images, the location of typical MS plaques (less than two spinal segments in length and less than half the cross-sectional area of the cord) is usually posterior or posterolateral, and they involve peripherally located white matter. The posterolateral location of the enhancing portion of the cord lesion on the postcontrast T1-weighted images in this patient could raise suspicion that it is an acute MS plaque rather than a neoplastic or infectious process. The constellation of imaging findings and the clinical features, however, appeared to favor neoplasm, and biopsy was performed.

Diffuse signal abnormalities of the cord on long TR images are not uncommon, and Lycklama a Nijeholt and colleagues reported that diffuse lesions were observed in approximately half as many patients with MS as were focal abnormalities. The diffuse abnormalities, however, were significantly associated with cervical cord atrophy (and the progressive subtypes of MS), not the cord enlargement seen in this case.

Notes

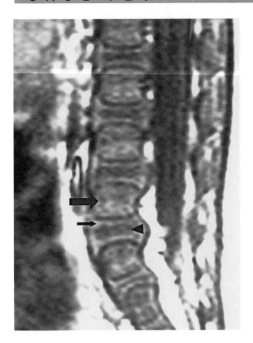
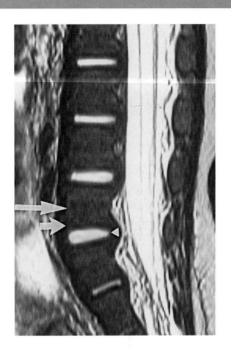

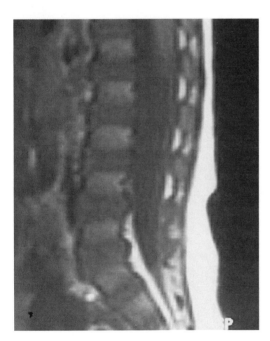

1. The two T1-weighted images were obtained from different patients. Which patient is younger?

2. The *large arrow*, *small arrow*, and *arrowhead* on the T1-weighted image (left) point to which structures?

3. Which structures enhance prominently in children younger than 18 months?

4. What explains a "pseudodisk" appearance on T1-weighted sagittal images?

Pediatric Spine, Normal MR Signal Intensities

1. The T1-weighted image on the left, with an accompanying T2-weighted fast-spin-echo image (center), was obtained from a 4-month-old, whereas the other T1-weighted image (right) was obtained from an 11-month-old.

2. Vertebral ossification center *(large arrow),* adjacent cartilage *(small arrow),* disk *(arrowhead).*

3. Ossification centers and cartilaginous end-plates.

4. When the cartilaginous end-plates and true disk are isointense, they produce the appearance of a single thick "disk," which has been called a "pseudodisk." The pseudodisk appearance usually occurs in stages I and II (see Comment); however, the 11-month-old shown here has pseudodisks. The thickness of the true disk in this child is closer to the thickness shown on the T2-weighted image. In stages I, II, and III, true disks are better assessed on T2-weighted images.

Reference

Sze G, Baierl P, Bravo S: Evolution of the infant spinal column: Evaluation with MR imaging. *Radiology* 181:819–827, 1991.

Cross-Reference

Neuroradiology: THE REQUISITES, pp 448–451.

Comment

The changing MR appearance of the normal spine in infants and children may be roughly separated into three stages, as proposed by Sze and colleagues. The signal intensities of the vertebral ossification center, adjacent cartilage, and disk are expressed relative to those of muscle on T1- and T2-weighted images.

On T1-weighted images, the progression is as follows:

• Stage I (birth to 1 month)—markedly hypointense ossification center, markedly hyperintense cartilage, isointense disk.

• Stage II (1 to 6 months)—the ossification center has hyperintense superior and inferior aspects (the inferior aspect is more hyperintense than the superior in the 4-month-old child shown here) and a hypointense center, with hyperintense cartilage and an isointense disk.

• Stage III (7 months to 2 years)—hyperintense ossification center, isointense cartilage, isointense disk (example of the 11-month-old shown here).

On T2-weighted images, the progression is as follows:

• Stage I—markedly hypointense ossification center, mildly hyperintense cartilage, markedly hyperintense disk.

• Stage II—the ossification center has an isointense to hypointense central portion *(large arrow)* with superior and inferior aspects that are isointense to hyperintense (relatively uniform signal throughout the ossification center is shown here), plus isointense to mildly hyperintense cartilage *(small arrow)* and a markedly hyperintense disk *(arrowhead).*

• Stage III—mildly hyperintense ossification center, isointense to mildly hyperintense cartilage, markedly hyperintense disk.

Notes

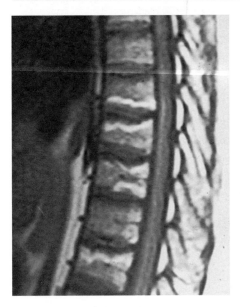
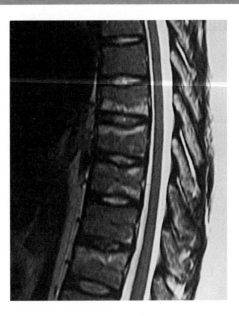

1. Are the abnormal vertebral signal intensities more likely due to acute or chronic changes?

2. How do the findings differ from those typically associated with type II end-plate changes?

3. What are the indications for percutaneous vertebroplasty?

4. Is osteoporosis better detected on a diffusion-weighted MR scan or on a CT scan?

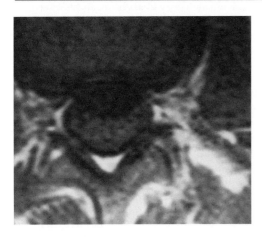
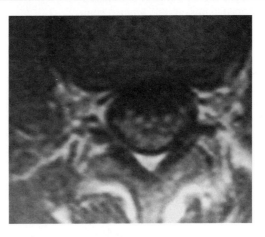

1. List five nonneoplastic conditions that may produce the features shown on the precontrast and postcontrast T1-weighted images (L1-2 level) in this patient with polyradiculoneuropathy.

2. Is the patient more likely to have diabetic amyotrophy or cytomegalovirus (CMV) infection?

3. Which is more likely to show cauda equina nerve root enhancement in adults, Charcot-Marie-Tooth disease (type I) or chronic inflammatory demyelinating polyradiculoneuropathy (CIDP)?

4. How does CIDP differ clinically from Guillain-Barré syndrome (GBS)?

Steroid-Induced, Chronic Osteoporotic Compression Fractures

1. Chronic.

2. The involved vertebrae have wedge-shaped (compression) deformities, whereas the adjacent disk spaces have approximately normal height and mild to moderate loss of signal intensity on the T2-weighted images. No appreciable osteophyte formation is present.

3. Percutaneous vertebroplasty is used for the treatment of destabilizing and painful vertebral lesions: osteoporotic compression fractures (age-related or steroid-induced vertebral collapse), vertebral hemangiomas, and malignant vertebral tumors (osteolytic metastases and multiple myeloma).

4. CT scan.

Reference

Baker LL, Goodman SB, Perkash I, Lane B, Enzmann DR: Benign versus pathologic compression fractures of vertebral bodies: Assessment with conventional spin-echo, chemical-shift, and STIR MR imaging. *Radiology* 174:495–502, 1990.

Cross-Reference

Neuroradiology: THE REQUISITES, pp 500–501.

Comment

This 21-year-old man with a history of long-term corticosteroid therapy for systemic lupus erythematosus underwent imaging because of a recent fall. Radiographs of the lumbar spine revealed diffuse osteopenia and a compression fracture of L1. On the T1-weighted and fast-spin-echo T2-weighted images, the T7, T8, T9, and T11 vertebrae have loss of stature and irregular bands of increased signal intensity involving the superior and inferior end-plates. The increased signal could represent either chronic, focal fatty marrow replacement or subacute hemorrhage. The presence of chemical shift effects (prominent dark zones superior to each of the bright bands at the superior end-plates), which are better seen on the T1-weighted image, indicates that the hyperintense bands represent fatty marrow accumulation and are therefore chronic. These findings are not typical of chronic benign compression fractures. Baker and colleagues found that chronic benign fractures usually demonstrated a marrow signal that was isointense relative to normal vertebrae on all pulse sequences. Only in about 10% of chronic benign fractures was high signal intensity observed.

None of the vertebrae shown here have low signal intensity on the T1-weighted image and high signal intensity on the T2-weighted image, as occurs in acute benign fractures and in pathologic fractures. If such features are present, diffusion-weighted and fat-saturated postcontrast T1-weighted MR images should also be obtained because they may help differentiate between benign and pathologic fractures. Pathologic fractures are more likely to show evidence of restricted diffusion and diffuse vertebral body enhancement, in addition to features of cortical destruction, involvement of posterior elements, and signal abnormalities of nonfractured vertebrae.

Notes

Chronic Inflammatory Demyelinating Polyradiculoneuropathy

1. GBS, CIDP, sarcoidosis, postradiation injury, and CMV infection.

2. CMV infection.

3. CIDP.

4. CIDP shows a chronic, often relapsing course (developing over months rather than weeks, as seen in GBS), pronounced sensory involvement, and responsiveness to corticosteroids—features lacking in GBS.

References

Dalakas MC: Advances in chronic inflammatory demyelinating polyneuropathy. *Curr Opin Neurol* 12:403–409, 1999.

Midroni G, de Tilly LN, Gray B, Vajsar J: MRI of the cauda equina in CIDP: Clinical correlations. *J Neurol Sci* 170:36–44, 1999.

Cross-Reference

Neuroradiology: THE REQUISITES, pp 478, 482, 487.

Comment

The precontrast and postcontrast images demonstrate enhancement of multiple spinal nerve roots in the cauda equina. They are not grossly enlarged or obviously clumped together. This 51-year-old man had a clinical course consistent with CIDP: a subacute onset and fluctuation of symptoms for many months. Spinal nerve (cauda equina) biopsy revealed demyelination and slight inflammatory changes. In the MR imaging study of CIDP referenced above, 69% (11 of 16) of patients with CIDP showed intrathecal nerve root enhancement (linear and diffuse) on postcontrast T1-weighted images, whereas none of the 15 controls (which included 5 patients with Charcot-Marie-Tooth disease, hereditary motor and sensory neuropathy [HMSN] type I) showed enhancement. Spinal nerve root enhancement has also been observed in GBS, with a frequency of up to 80% to 95% of patients in some studies. Enlargement of nerve roots is not a feature of GBS and occurs uncommonly in CIDP.

In addition to the conditions listed in answer 1 above, intrathecal nerve root enhancement as shown here may be observed in cases of polyradiculopathy secondary to multilevel degenerative spine disease, infectious (pyogenic or granulomatous) disease, or neoplastic disease involving the leptomeninges (carcinomatosis, lymphoma, leukemia). Interestingly, in the referenced study one patient with CIDP had a combination of linear and nodular enhancement throughout the cauda equina. Nerve root enhancement is not a feature of diabetic polyradiculoneuropathy (diabetic amyotrophy), which may mimic CIDP clinically.

The immunopathogenesis of CIDP is not fully understood, yet alteration of the blood-nerve barrier (BNB), possibly allowing nerve root enhancement on MR imaging studies, has been proposed as a fundamental event in the development of inflammatory demyelinating neuropathies. After breaching the BNB, macrophages and T cells enter the endoneurium and initiate a cascade of reactions involving antimyelin antibodies and multiple other cellular elements that cause demyelination, as well as axonal loss.

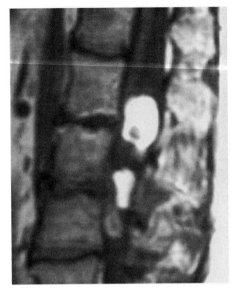
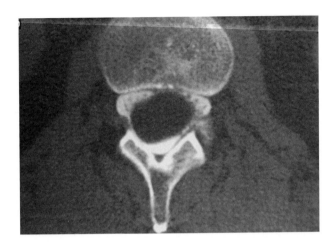

1. Based on the sagittal T1-weighted image and the axial CT myelogram (L1-2 level), is the rounded L1-2 lesion primarily intramedullary, intradural extramedullary, or extradural?

2. List three tumors that may have this appearance.

3. Which findings on MR imaging or CT can help narrow the differential diagnosis?

4. This patient is potentially at increased risk of meningitis from what two sources?

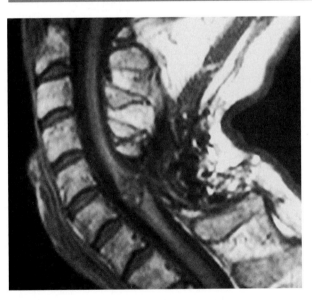
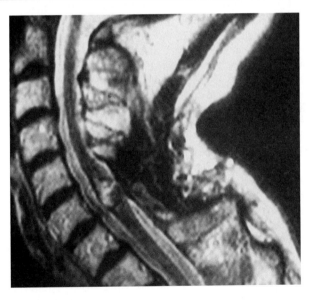

1. This 60-year-old man was clinically stable for 7 years after excision of a spinal arteriovenous malformation (AVM). List four potential causes for recent progression of his myelopathy over 3 years.

2. What additional MR imaging studies may be helpful in distinguishing among the potential causes?

3. Which is more difficult to treat, a type I or type II AVM?

4. Which have a greater rate of recurrence of hemorrhage if untreated—spinal cord or cerebral AVMs?

Intradural, Cystic Teratoma

1. At surgery the mass had both intramedullary and extramedullary components.

2. Dermoid, lipoma, and teratoma.

3. A combination of lipid and cystic/gelatinous components (better seen on MR imaging than CT) favors dermoid or teratoma over lipoma. The presence of coarse calcification or teeth (better shown on CT) favors teratoma.

4. Dermoid or teratoma can produce a chemical meningitis after rupture. A dorsal dermal sinus, which is found in association with approximately 20% to 25% of spinal dermoids, increases the risk of infectious meningitis.

Reference

Mhatre P, Hudgins PA, Hunter S: Dermoid cyst in the lumbosacral region: Radiographic findings. *AJR Am J Roentgenol* 174:874–875, 2000.

Cross-Reference

Neuroradiology: THE REQUISITES, p 484.

Comment

The MR image shows two areas in the lumbar canal that are hyperintense to muscle and isointense to fat. The area at L1-2 has a small region of lower signal intensity, representing a cyst, whereas the area at L2-3 is homogeneous. These hyperintense areas may result from the presence of lipid, hemorrhage (subacute), or iophendylate (Pantopaque) accumulation. The CT myelogram shows that the area at L1-2 has the density of lipid, consistent with dermoid, lipoma, or teratoma. CT also demonstrates multiple roots of the cauda equina surrounded by contrast material in the subarachnoid space anterior to the intradural mass. The central portion of the cauda equina is contiguous with the anterior surface of the mass at L1-2. At surgery, gelatinous regions were found interspersed with areas of adipose tissue along the filum terminale, which resulted in an elongated mass of mixed consistency (and heterogeneous signal) between L1 and L3. The filum was tethered to the inferior portion of the mass. The final diagnosis was benign cystic teratoma, with squamous mucosa, subcutaneous glands, and predominantly adipose tissue seen on histopathologic examination.

Teratomas are extremely rare within the CNS, where they account for only about 0.1% of primary intracranial tumors. With the exception of sacrococcygeal teratomas, which are relatively frequent, teratomas within the spinal canal are rarer than intracranial teratomas. Intraspinal teratomas are associated with spina bifida. The tumors are composed of derivatives of the three primitive germ cell layers and may thus have epidermal, dermal, adipose, vascular, cartilaginous, and muscular elements. By comparison, dermoids are unilocular or multilocular cystic masses lined by simple or stratified squamous epithelium with an underlying layer similar to dermis; this layer may contain hair follicles, sweat glands, and sebaceous glands. The hyperintensity of dermoids on T1-weighted images has been attributed to the secretions of sebaceous glands, liquid lipid metabolites, and/or cholesterol from decomposed epithelial cells of the cyst wall.

Postoperative Cord Tethering, Cervical

1. Recurrent AVM with a steal phenomenon, development of a syrinx, cord tethering, and slow, ongoing hemorrhage from a residual AVM.

2. CSF flow-sensitive sequences, contrast-enhanced MR imaging, and MR angiography.

3. Type II.

4. Spinal cord AVMs.

References

Detweiler PW, Porter RW, Spetzler RF: Spinal arteriovenous malformations. *Neurosurg Clin N Am* 10:89–100, 1999.
Niimi Y, Berenstein A: Endovascular treatment of spinal vascular malformations. *Neurosurg Clin N Am* 10:47–71, 1999.

Cross-Reference

Neuroradiology: THE REQUISITES, pp 496–498.

Comment

The patient has evidence of previous C5 through C7 laminectomies. At C6 the cord is focally enlarged and has inhomogeneous signal intensity. In the inferoposterior part of the lesion is an area of intermediate/low signal intensity on the T1-weighted image and low signal intensity on the T2-weighted image, consistent with acute or chronic hemorrhage. The larger anterosuperior part of the lesion has high signal intensity on the T2-weighted image, consistent with myelomalacia or possibly edema. No area of CSF-equivalent signal intensity can be seen in the cord, and therefore no macroscopic intramedullary cyst (i.e., no syrinx) is present. The punctate foci of high signal intensity on the T1-weighted images are probably due to paramagnetic effects from subacute hemorrhage. On the T2-weighted image, CSF signal intensity posterior to the cord at C6 is absent, and the cord surface appears to be contiguous with the dural surface, suggestive of tethering. This region failed to show any evidence of CSF motion on MR flow images. No serpentine flow voids are seen on the T2-weighted image, and contrast-enhanced three-dimensional MR angiography failed to show any abnormally enlarged or tortuous intradural veins, as would be expected for a recurrent/residual spinal AVM. The patient's new clinical symptoms were therefore attributed to a tethered cord and progressive myelomalacic myelopathy. His symptoms improved after untethering of the cord, lysis of nerve root adhesions, and expansile duraplasty with freeze-dried dural allograft.

This patient was originally treated for a glomus-type AVM of the cervical cord. Although these AVMs may be treated solely by endovascular techniques, the rate of complete obliteration is relatively low in comparison with the rate for spinal cord arteriovenous fistulas. Thus, treatment usually involves preoperative embolization, especially of associated aneurysms, to reduce the risk of hemorrhage, followed by complete surgical resection of the AVM nidus. A potential complication of surgery, as shown here, is the delayed development of cord tethering and adhesions, without a syrinx.

Notes

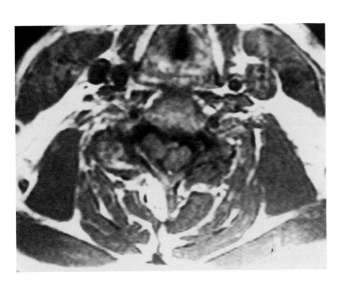
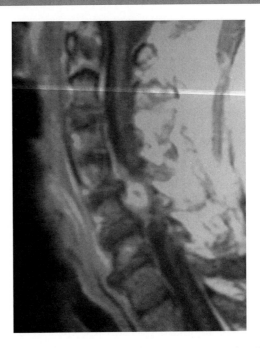

1. Name three neoplasms that may produce the features visible on the axial T1-weighted image (C5 level) and the right parasagittal postcontrast T1-weighted image.

2. Name three nonneoplastic lesions that may also produce the MR features.

3. Does the presence of a "dural tail" sign favor a neoplastic or nonneoplastic etiology?

4. Is "sequestered" disk the same as "uncontained" disk? "migrated" disk?

Disk Herniation (Sequestration), Cervical

1. Schwannoma, meningioma, and lymphoma.

2. Sequestered disk fragment, epidural abscess, and synovial cyst.

3. The "dural tail," which is a region of dural enhancement that trails off with distance from the lesion, is often a sign of a meningioma; however, any process (neoplastic or inflammatory) that involves the dura may produce this sign.

4. No. No.

Reference

Ross JS, Modic MT, Masaryk TJ, Carter J, Marcus RE, Bohlman H: Assessment of extradural degenerative disease with Gd-DTPA–enhanced MR imaging: Correlation with surgical and pathologic findings. *AJR Am J Roentgenol* 154:151–157, 1990.

Cross-Reference

Neuroradiology: THE REQUISITES, pp 461–463, 514.

Comment

The axial image shows a C5 right-sided extradural mass with a linear extension or tail coursing medially. On the postcontrast parasagittal image the mass has a central nonenhancing area surrounded by thick peripheral enhancement that is continuous with adjacent, less intense epidural enhancement. There appears to be a disk herniation at C4-5, although it is not continuous with the nonenhancing area within the mass. The differential diagnosis includes meningioma, which usually enhances homogeneously, and schwannoma, which may have nonenhancing cystic areas. Epidural abscess is likely to involve more vertebral segments and, when anteriorly located, to be associated with diskitis/osteomyelitis. A synovial cyst must be considered because of the proximity of the mass to the right lamina and facet complex on the axial image, although the postcontrast enhancement is quite prominent for a typical synovial cyst. The patient went to surgery with a preliminary diagnosis of spinal tumor. Pathologically, the resected mass was composed of dense connective tissue, fibrocartilage, cartilage, bone fragments, and a mesenchymal reaction. No tumor was detected.

Although more commonly seen in the lumbar spine, sequestered disk fragments may also be observed in the cervical spine. The nonenhancing center of the mass at C5 is the sequestered or "free" fragment. By definition, this fragment is not in continuity with the parent herniated disk at C4-5. The enhancement is due to the vascular fibrous (scar) tissue that surrounds the fragment, as well as the accumulation of contrast in the adjacent epidural venous plexus. Ross and colleagues have observed that peridiskal scar tissue in unoperated patients is histologically identical to the epidural scar tissue seen postoperatively.

An "uncontained" herniated disk, which is a herniation through a disrupted outer anulus fibrosus, may or may not be in continuity with the disk space of origin. Thus, the term "uncontained" is not synonymous with "sequestered." The term "migrated" refers to the position of herniated disk material relative to the disk space of origin and does not specify whether the disk material is continuous or discontinuous with that disk space. Hence, "migrated" is also not synonymous with "sequestered." In this case the sequestered disk fragment has migrated (i.e., been displaced) caudad.

Notes

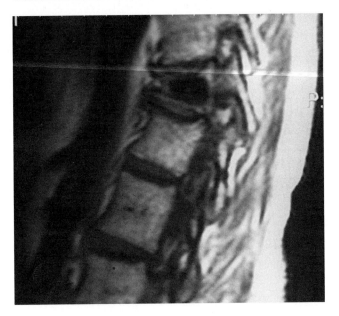
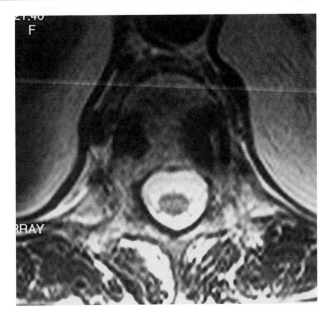

1. List four conditions that can produce marked hypointensity within a vertebra on all MR images.
2. What is the principal mechanism of signal loss in the T11 vertebra?
3. What is the most likely cause of the T11 fracture?
4. How would one expect these lesions to appear on plain radiographs, and why?

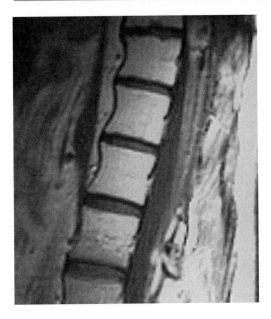
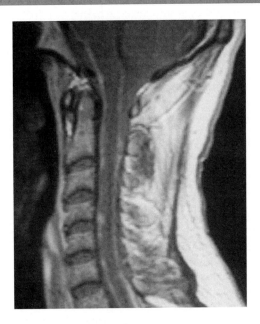

1. List five nonneoplastic, noninfectious causes of leptomeningeal enhancement.
2. The postcontrast T1-weighted images were obtained approximately 1 year apart. Is the enhancement in the cervical spine more likely to be due to neoplastic, inflammatory, or vascular disease? Why?
3. List three primary pigmented tumors of the leptomeninges.
4. Are intracranial ependymomas more likely than spinal ependymomas to disseminate?

Percutaneous Vertebroplasty

1. Fracture with compaction of dense bone, osteoblastic metastases, type III degenerative end-plate changes, and foreign body (bullet, polymethylmethacrylate [PMMA]).

2. Extremely short proton T2 relaxation times for the solid, polymerized methylmethacrylate.

3. Osteoporosis.

4. Hyperdense because the injected PMMA paste contains radiopaque barium sulfate and tantalum or tungsten powder.

References

Deramond H, Depriester C, Galibert P, Le Gars D: Percutaneous vertebroplasty with polymethylmethacrylate. *Radiol Clin North Am* 36:533-546, 1998.

Jensen ME, Evans AJ, Mathis JM, Kallmes DF, Cloft HJ, Dion JE: Percutaneous polymethylmethacrylate vertebroplasty in the treatment of osteoporotic vertebral body compression fractures: Technical aspects. *AJNR Am J Neuroradiol* 18:1897-1904, 1997.

Cross-Reference

Neuroradiology: THE REQUISITES, pp 493, 500.

Comment

On the sagittal T1-weighted image is seen a wedge-shaped compression fracture of the T11 body, and most of the body is markedly hypointense. The axial fast-spin-echo T2-weighted image of T11 shows that the vertebral body actually has bilateral areas of hypointensity, as well as hypointensity in the right paraspinal soft tissues. The posterior cortex at the level of the pedicles is disrupted. These findings should alert the reader to the possibility of an "implanted" foreign body, namely, PMMA, that has been introduced into the vertebral body via a percutaneous transpediculate approach. The procedure, referred to as percutaneous vertebroplasty or simply vertebroplasty, is used to treat destabilizing and painful vertebral lesions: osteoporotic compression fractures, vertebral hemangiomas, and malignant vertebral tumors (osteolytic metastases and multiple myeloma). The case shown here does not have any obvious evidence of a vertebral hemangioma or malignant tumor, so the most likely cause of the T11 fracture is osteoporosis.

The vertebroplasty technique in the thoracic and lumbar regions involves puncture of a pedicle and injection of the polymerizing PMMA into the vertebral body. When less than 50% of the body is filled by the injection, as in this case, a contralateral puncture with injection of additional PMMA may be performed to better maintain the vertebral stature. The principal risk of this technique is leakage of PMMA into the paravertebral soft tissues (as seen on the right in this case), the spinal canal or neural foramina, adjacent disks, or the epidural veins. Some authors recommend performing venography before injection of the polymer mixture. In patients with malignant neoplasms, radiation therapy is performed after vertebroplasty. The two treatments complement each other with respect to analgesic effect.

Notes

CNS Dissemination of Conus Ependymoma

1. Subarachnoid hemorrhage, postsurgical changes, radiation therapy, intrathecal chemotherapy, and spontaneous intracranial hypotension. Another cause is sarcoidosis.

2. Neoplastic leptomeningeal disease is favored because of the peripheral, nodular enhancement pattern within the cervical canal and the evidence of previous radiation therapy and surgery at the thoracolumbar junction.

3. Pigmented meningioma, malignant melanoma, and meningeal melanocytoma. Also included are melanotic schwannoma and meningeal melanocytoma.

4. No.

Reference

Rezai AR, Woo HH, Lee M, Cohen H, Zagzag D, Epstein FJ: Disseminated ependymomas of the central nervous system. *J Neurosurg* 85:618-624, 1996.

Cross-Reference

Neuroradiology: THE REQUISITES, pp 487-489.

Comment

The postcontrast image of the thoracolumbar spine shows evidence of laminectomies from L1 to at least the level of T11 (uppermost vertebral body). Although we have no precontrast image for comparison, there is inhomogeneous enhancement of the conus medullaris and cauda equina, with a conus mass at the upper edge of the figure. The bodies of T11 through L2 demonstrate marked hyperintensity compatible with postradiation changes. The cervical spine MR image, obtained 1 year later, demonstrates leptomeningeal enhancement, with multiple nodular foci extending from the cervical region to the basal cisterns of the posterior fossa and apparent tonsillar ectopia. No radiation changes can be seen in the cervical vertebrae. The combination of findings on the two images should suggest to the reader that this patient has leptomeningeal metastatic disease, probably secondary to CSF spread of metastases from a conus tumor (most commonly an ependymoma) that was incompletely resected and therefore received postoperative radiation therapy.

The goal of surgical treatment of both intracranial and spinal ependymomas is gross total resection. The extent of the initial resection is highly significant with respect to subsequent dissemination. Rezai and colleagues found that disseminated disease never developed in about 80% of patients with total resection, whereas about 70% of patients with subtotal resection demonstrated dissemination (although the method used to determine dissemination was not elucidated in their article). The incidence of dissemination for primary spinal ependymomas was 12.5%, versus 9.6% for primary intracranial ependymomas. Most of the disseminated tumors from primary spinal lesions were of the myxopapillary histologic subtype. This subtype is commonly found in primary ependymomas of the filum terminale, cauda equina, or conus (as in this case).

Notes

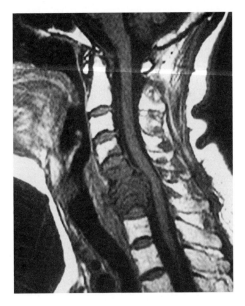
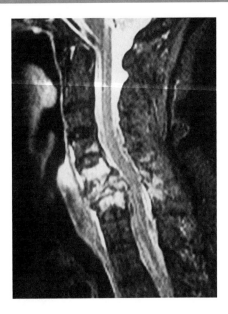

1. Is this condition more likely to be infection or tumor?

2. What are the most common granulomatous infections of the spine?

3. List three nonneoplastic conditions that mimic infectious diskitis/osteomyelitis on CT but can often be distinguished on MR imaging. What are the distinguishing features on MR imaging?

4. In general, what two imaging findings tend to favor metastatic disease over osteomyelitis?

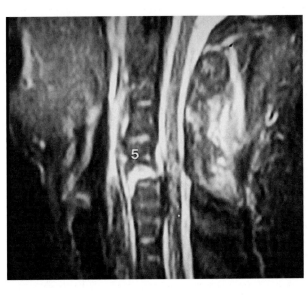
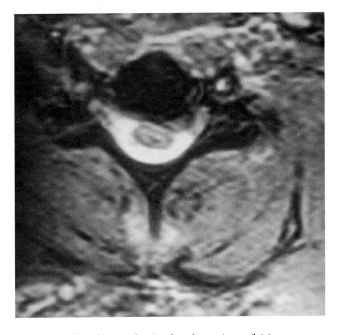

1. Is MR imaging likely to be more or less sensitive than conventional radiography in the detection of (a) acute fracture, (b) acute facet subluxation or dislocation, and (c) canal stenosis?

2. Based on the sagittal and axial (C6-7 level) images, would you favor a one- or two-level anterior cervical diskectomy and fusion?

3. What is the condition of the anterior longitudinal ligament?

4. What MR imaging findings help differentiate bilateral from unilateral facet dislocation?

Metastasis Mimicking Diskitis/Osteomyelitis

1. A diagnosis of tumor is more likely because of the radiation changes in the upper cervical vertebral bodies. Tumor and infection may be indistinguishable, however, and biopsy is needed for diagnosis and treatment.

2. Tuberculosis, brucellosis, and fungal infections (blastomycosis, cryptococcosis, and coccidioidomycosis).

3. Renal spondyloarthropathy associated with long-term hemodialysis; spinal neuroarthropathy associated with tabes dorsalis, syringomyelia, and diabetes mellitus; and severe degenerative disease. The distinguishing features are the relatively decreased signal intensity within the involved disk space and, often, the adjacent vertebral bodies on T2-weighted images.

4. Involvement of the pedicles and sparing of the intervertebral disks.

References

Kim JK, Ryu KN, Choi WS, Choe BK, Choi JM, Yoon AY: Spinal involvement of hematopoietic malignancies and metastasis: Differentiation using MR imaging. *Clin Imaging* 23:125–133, 1999.

Park YH, Taylor JA, Szollar SM, Resnick D: Imaging findings in spinal neuroarthropathy. *Spine* 19:1499-1504, 1994.

Cross-Reference

Neuroradiology: THE REQUISITES, pp 477–478, 491.

Comment

The MR images show destruction of C5 through C7, with epidural and prevertebral extension. The findings are compatible with diskitis/osteomyelitis: (1) confluent, decreased signal and an inability to discern a cortical margin between the endplates and the disk on the T1-weighted image, (2) increased signal intensity within the presumed intervertebral disks and within the adjacent vertebral bodies on the T2-weighted image, and (3) prominent paravertebral masses and prevertebral extension of disease.

These findings are also compatible with a neoplastic process. The hyperintensity (radiation changes) in the intact cervical vertebrae plus involvement of the posterior elements of C5 through C7 support a diagnosis of neoplasm. In adults, extension of osteomyelitis from the vertebral bodies into the posterior neural arch occurs in approximately ≤12% of cases. By comparison, Kim and colleagues found that metastases involved the anterior and posterior elements in 76% of cases and the anterior element (body and/or pedicle) alone in 24% of cases. Hematopoietic malignancies (lymphoma, leukemia, multiple myeloma) involved the anterior and posterior elements in 100% of cases.

Among tumors, metastases are the most common mimickers of diskitis/osteomyelitis. Less common are primary bone tumors, such as plasmacytoma, eosinophilic granuloma, aneurysmal bone cyst, giant cell tumor, and chordoma.

The type I pattern of degenerative changes in the vertebral body marrow ("end-plate" changes) on MR imaging (low on T1-weighted and high on T2-weighted images) parallels the changes occurring in osteomyelitis; however, the signal intensity of the disk on T2-weighted images is usually decreased in degenerative disease and increased in diskitis.

Traumatic Disk Herniation, Cervical

1. (a) Similar, (b) less, and (c) more—based on the results of a recent prospective study (58 patients with 172 acute cervical injuries) by Katzberg and colleagues with an open-design 0.3-tesla scanner.

2. Two-level, because of the necessity for diskectomies at both C5-6 and C6-7.

3. Intact.

4. Greater than 50% anterior subluxation or translation of the vertebral body above a ruptured disk relative to the vertebral body below the disk favors bilateral facet dislocation. Rotation of the vertebra above the level of the disk disruption relative to the vertebra below it favors unilateral facet dislocation.

References

Bucciero A, Carangelo B, Cerillo A, Gammone V, Panagiotopoulos K, Vizioli L: Myeloradicular damage in traumatic cervical disc herniation. *J Neurosurg Sci* 42:203–211, 1998.

Katzberg RW, Benedetti PF, Drake CM, et al: Acute cervical spine injuries: Prospective MR imaging assessment at a level 1 trauma center. *Radiology* 213:203–212, 1999.

Cross-Reference

Neuroradiology: THE REQUISITES, pp 498–499.

Comment

The sagittal STIR (short tau inversion recovery) T2-weighted image shows a ruptured disk at C5-6 and grade 1 (<25% anteroposterior diameter of the vertebral body) anterosubluxation of C5 on C6. The low signal intensity posterior to the C6 body is due to acute epidural hematoma and fragmented disk material (operative findings). Although the anterior displacement of C5 on C6 is less than 50% of the C6 body, bilateral facet dislocation was present, and it was reduced at surgery. The axial gradient-echo T2*-weighted image shown here is at the C6-7 level, where a herniated disk projects into the medial aspect of the left neural foramen. This traumatic herniation is also seen on the sagittal image and appears to compress the cord. This finding must be recognized and reported so that if surgical treatment requiring an anterior cervical diskectomy and fusion (ACDF) is planned, it should include both C5-6 and C6-7 disk levels (two-level ACDF). The increased signal intensity within the cord on both the T2- and T2*-weighted images is consistent with the presence of edema.

In their prospective study comparing MR with conventional radiographs in the detection of acute cervical spine injuries, Katzberg and associates found that 43% of acute fractures and 59% of acute facet subluxations/dislocations were detected on MR images as compared with 48% and 72%, respectively, on conventional radiographs. MR imaging was significantly better in demonstrating chronic underlying canal stenosis in the population studied. In a study of pure traumatic cervical disk herniations in 41 patients, Bucciero and colleagues found that the most common level was C5-6, with 58.5%, versus 19.5% at C6-7, 17.1% at C4-5, and 9.7% at C3-4.

Notes

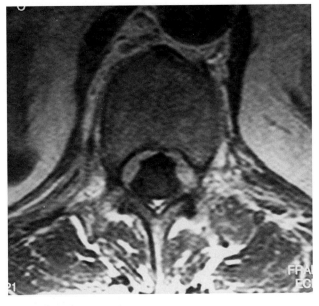

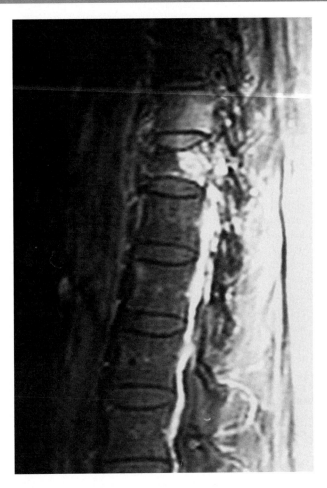

1. Identify the enhancing structures located anteriorly and laterally in the spinal canal on the postcontrast T1-weighted axial (T12 level) and fat-saturated sagittal images.

2. What is their function?

3. Name the two types of metastases based on hematogenous spread, and their likely vertebral locations.

4. List the four major components of the vertebral venous plexus.

Vertebral Lymphoma With Secondary Epidural Venous Enlargement

1. Engorged anterior internal (epidural) veins.

2. To drain blood from the vertebrae and the epidural tissues (fat, muscle).

3. Arterial metastases tend to lodge in the end arterioles and sinusoids adjacent to the vertebral end-plates. Venous metastases, which reach the vertebra by retrograde flow in the epidural venous plexus, would hypothetically be found in the posterior central portion of the vertebral body near the basivertebral vein. Experimental and clinical evidence indicates that the pattern of vertebral metastases is more complicated than passive hemodynamics. In part, it also depends on the interaction of a particular tumor type (e.g., breast, prostate, lung) with the microenvironment of the "target" tissue ("seed and soil" hypothesis).

4. Internal vertebral veins, anterior and posterior plexuses; external vertebral veins, anterior and posterior plexuses; basivertebral vein and plexus; and intervertebral veins.

References

Arguello F, Baggs RB, Duerst RE, Johnstone L, McQueen K, Frantz CN: Pathogenesis of vertebral metastasis and epidural spinal cord compression. *Cancer* 65:98–106, 1990.

Yuh WT, Quets JP, Lee HJ, et al: Anatomic distribution of metastases in the vertebral body and modes of hematogenous spread. *Spine* 21:2243–2250, 1996.

Cross-Reference

Neuroradiology: THE REQUISITES, pp 449–451.

Comment

This 70-year-old man had a 2-month history of back pain. The left parasagittal image demonstrates a pathologic compression fracture of T11 with abnormal enhancement within the posterior portions of the bodies of T10 and T11. Retropulsion of the posterior portion of T11 into the canal is difficult to detect on the parasagittal image. The epidural enhancement is striking and confluent and follows the course of the internal vertebral venous plexus from T11 to the lumbar region. The axial image at the T12 level shows bilateral, symmetric enhancing "masses" in the anterior epidural space. Given the epidural venous enhancement pattern on the parasagittal image, the "masses" at T12 most likely represent engorged anterior internal epidural veins. The enlarged veins below T11 are the result of (1) compression of the anterior venous plexus by tumor or displaced bone at T11 and/or (2) intravenous tumor or thrombosis at T11. Biopsy of T11 revealed B-cell lymphoma. Whereas diffuse multilevel marrow involvement by lymphoma could account for the lesion in the body at T10, the posterior location suggests that lymphoma may have spread locally via the vertebral venous plexuses from T11.

The vertebral venous system is a valveless anastomotic system in which blood flows either cephalad or caudad, depending on changes in intrathoracic and intraabdominal (respiration, coughing) pressure and hydrostatic (changes in posture) factors. The anterior internal vertebral venous plexus has a relatively constant morphologic pattern consisting of a pair of longitudinal trunks (one left and one right) located anterolaterally in the canal. Some authors divide each trunk into medial and lateral veins. The trunks deviate laterally at the level of the intervertebral disk and converge medially at the midpoint of the vertebral body, where they unite with the basivertebral vein. The trunks are located anterior to the posterior longitudinal ligament (PLL) at the level of the vertebral body and then posterior to the PLL where it merges with the intervertebral disk. Normally, the size of the anterior internal vertebral plexus gradually increases from C1 down to L5 and rapidly decreases in the sacral canal. This variation may be due to a corresponding increase in vertebral body volume (greatest in the lumbar region) and associated increased drainage from the basivertebral vein into the anterior internal veins. When compared with the anterior internal vertebral venous plexus, the posterior internal plexus is less constant and shows segmental and interindividual differences. It is more difficult to opacify on radiologic and anatomic studies and is routinely smaller. Anastomoses between the anterior and posterior internal plexuses at each vertebral level and between the internal and external venous plexuses have been described.

Notes

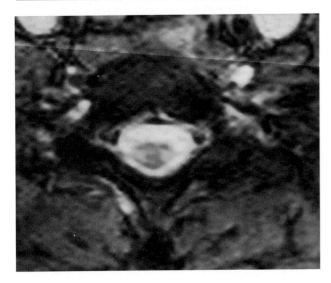

1. List three conditions that may produce the findings shown on this gradient-echo image (C7 level).

2. Why is this condition unlikely to be arterial or venous infarction?

3. Are the majority of spinal cord MS plaques found in the cervical or thoracic cord?

4. In diffusion-weighted imaging of the spinal cord, name two measurable properties of white matter that are likely to be altered when demyelination and axonal loss are present.

Multiple Sclerosis, Cervical

1. Amyotrophic lateral sclerosis, multiple sclerosis (MS), and traumatic cord injury above the C7 level with antegrade wallerian degeneration.

2. Arterial infarction usually involves the anterior two thirds of the cord, particularly the central gray matter (anterior spinal artery territory), which is spared in this case. Posterior spinal artery infarction is rare and tends to involve the posterior columns more than the lateral columns. Most documented cases of venous infarction result from venous congestion secondary to a dural arteriovenous fistula. The signal abnormality is patchy or diffuse and predominantly central rather than peripheral in location.

3. Cervical cord.

4. Mean diffusivity and anisotropy.

References

Clark CA, Werring DJ, Miller DH: Diffusion imaging of the spinal cord in vivo: Estimation of the principal diffusivities and application to multiple sclerosis. *Magn Reson Med* 43:133–138, 2000.

Cross-Reference

Neuroradiology: THE REQUISITES, pp 480–481.

Comment

The T2*-weighted axial image shows bilateral high signal intensity in the lateral columns (including the corticospinal, rubrospinal, and spinocerebellar white matter tracts). No cord enlargement is present, and the dorsal columns are relatively spared. The MS plaques in this patient mimic the appearance of conditions such as amyotrophic lateral sclerosis and spinal cord trauma that produce degeneration of the bilateral corticospinal tracts.

The white matter tracts in the spinal cord are predominantly longitudinally oriented structures that more or less restrict the movement of water molecules, depending on the direction of their average displacement. Thus, water molecules that diffuse parallel to the long axis of the tracts, that is, in approximately the supero-inferior direction, essentially move without restriction, whereas molecules that diffuse perpendicular to the long axis, namely, in the right-left or anteroposterior direction, have restricted motion. This phenomenon is referred to as diffusion anisotropy. If the fiber structure of the white matter is disrupted, for example, by demyelination and especially axonal loss, diffusion perpendicular to the long axis of the fibers becomes less restricted and anisotropy is diminished. In addition, less restricted motion in the right-left or anteroposterior direction results in an increase in mean diffusivity. Preliminary reports indicate that such changes are occurring in chronic MS plaques of the spinal cord. For acute inflammatory lesions, edema may contribute to the increased mean diffusivity and loss of anisotropy. Measures of white matter integrity based on diffusion-weighted MR imaging may prove to be more sensitive than standard spin-echo imaging of cord morphology based on T1 and T2 relaxation times and the spin density of water protons.

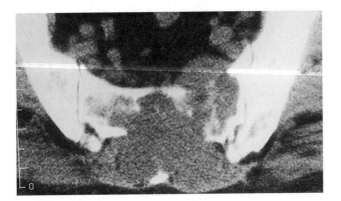
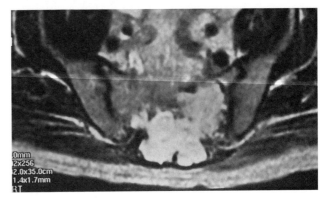
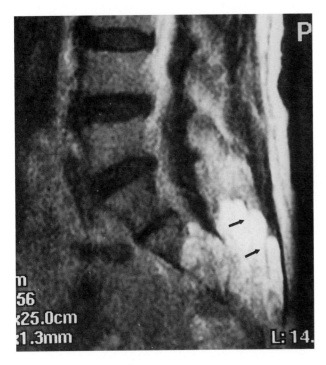

1. List five tumors that may have the appearance shown on the noncontrast CT image and T2-weighted axial and sagittal MR images from a 70-year-old man with back pain.

2. Which of these tumors favors a midline location?

3. What is a parachordoma?

4. What percentage of chordomas originate in the sacrococcygeal region?

Chordoma, Sacral

1. Metastatic carcinoma, lymphoma, plasmacytoma/myeloma, sarcoma, and chordoma.

2. Chordoma.

3. Parachordoma is a rare tumor composed of cells that are microscopically similar to fetal notochordal cells; however, a parachordoma has interstitial mucoid material with staining properties that differ from those of chordoma. Parachordomas involve the soft tissues adjacent to tendons, synovium, and bone.

4. 50%.

References

Coombs RJ, Coiner L: Sacral chordoma with unusual posterior radiographic presentation. *Skeletal Radiol* 25:679–681, 1996.

York JE, Kaczaraj A, Abi-Said D, et al: Sacral chordoma: 40-year experience at a major cancer center. *Neurosurgery* 44:74–79, 1999.

Cross-Reference

Neuroradiology: THE REQUISITES, p 494.

Comment

The CT image at the S2-3 level shows a soft tissue mass that appears to originate in the sacrum. Bone destruction can be seen in the midline extending to the posterior paraspinal muscles, as well as in the left sacral ala extending into the presacral region. On the corresponding T2-weighted MR image the mass is hyperintense. The findings are typical for a destructive neoplasm but are not specific, and several tumors may be considered in the differential diagnosis, as noted above. Two findings may help distinguish chordoma: a midline location and the presence of hypointense septations separating the hyperintense lobules that make up the bulk of the mass. In this case, some lobulations and septations (*arrows*) are seen on the sagittal image but not on the axial image.

Because they originate from notochordal remnants, chordomas may involve any segment of the craniospinal axis from the sphenoid to the coccyx. The approximate frequency of involvement is as follows: sacrococcygeal, 50%; clival, 35%; remainder of the spine, 15%. Sacral chordomas usually extend anteriorly and compress or invade the lower sacral nerves rather than extending posteriorly. Typical chordomas consist of mucin-containing physaliphorous cells and/or purely cystic mucinous pools, which account for the hyperintensity seen on T2-weighted images. The hypointense septations that are sometimes seen represent fibrous strands between the lobular components of the tumor.

Sacral chordomas are slow growing and relatively resistant to radiation and chemotherapy. Five- and 10-year survival rates are on the order of 50% and 30%, respectively. Radical resection is associated with a significantly longer disease-free interval than is subtotal removal of the tumor. The addition of radiation after subtotal resection improves the disease-free interval, but in general, radiotherapy can be used only once. Metastases occur in about one fourth of patients.

Notes

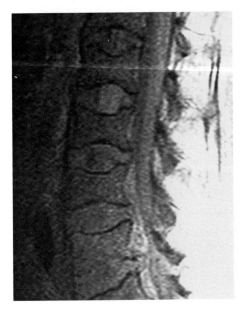
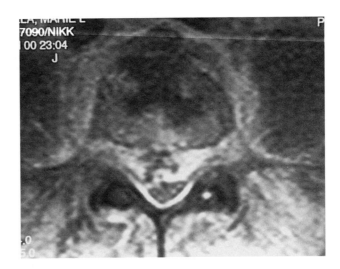

1. This 57-year-old black woman with fever had pain and tenderness at L4. Name the two most likely etiologies.
2. List four potential causes of myelopathy in patients with the disorder illustrated by this case.
3. Name five conditions in which vertebral biconcavity has been reported.
4. What animal has similarly shaped vertebral bodies?

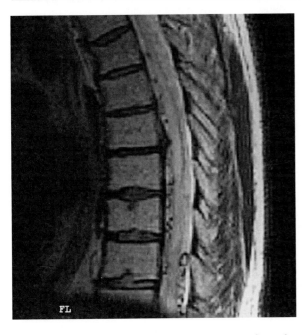
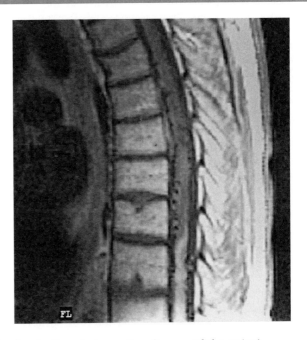

1. List at least four nonneoplastic causes of myelopathy (excluding degenerative disease of the spine).
2. Which of these causes is suggested by the T2-weighted and postcontrast T1-weighted images above?
3. Which of the MR imaging findings is likely to be most specific?
4. Why is cord enhancement seen on the T1-weighted image?

C A S E   1 3 3

Sickle Cell Disease With Infection

1. Bone infarction, infection, or both. Infection causing salmonella osteomyelitis occurs almost exclusively in patients with sickle cell disease.

2. Spinal cord infarction, epidural abscess, extramedullary hematopoiesis, and vertebral body infarction leading to collapse.

3. Sickle cell disease (Hb SS), thalassemia major, Gaucher's disease, hereditary spherocytosis, and homocystinuria.

4. Certain species of fish have a uniform biconcave contour of their vertebral bodies, hence the term "fish" vertebrae.

Reference

Martino AM, Winfield JA: *Salmonella* osteomyelitis with epidural abscess. A case report with review of osteomyelitis in children with sickle cell anemia. *Pediatr Neurosurg* 16:321–325, 1990.

Cross-Reference

Neuroradiology: THE REQUISITES, pp 477–482.

Comment

Sickle cell patients are more prone than others to certain infections, including pneumococcal and *Salmonella* infections, as a result of decreased phagocytic ability of the reticuloendothelial system. This patient had sepsis and meningitis attributable to *Streptococcus pneumoniae*. She had been treated with antibiotics for 12 days when MR images were obtained because of persistent fever and back pain. The fast-spin-echo proton-density-weighted image shows diffusely decreased signal intensity within the vertebral bodies relative to the disk spaces, consistent with bone marrow hyperplasia. The body of L4 is slightly hyperintense in comparison to the other vertebral bodies, and its inferior end-plate is indistinct—features suggestive of osteomyelitis. The adjacent disk space had a normal appearance on all other sequences. A variably hyperintense anterior epidural mass or collection extends from L3 through L5, with marked compression of the thecal sac and cauda equina at L4. On the postcontrast, fat-saturated T1-weighted axial image at L4 can be seen inhomogeneous enhancement within the L4 body and in the paravertebral and epidural spaces. An anterior epidural abscess was confirmed at surgery.

The skeletal imaging findings in sickle cell disease are due to (1) bone marrow hyperplasia secondary to anemia and (2) bone and marrow ischemia and infarction secondary to sickling episodes. In the spine the vertebral bodies have been described as having an H shape and/or a smoothly curved end-plate depression. The H vertebral body shape, an angulated depression of the central portion of the end-plate, has been attributed to a growth disturbance of the central area secondary to ischemia/infarction. Some authors distinguish this shape from a smoothly curved end-plate depression attributed to osteoporosis secondary to bone marrow hyperplasia. Other authors use the general term "biconcave" to refer to the vertebral end-plate contour abnormalities.

Notes

C A S E   1 3 4

Dural Arteriovenous Fistula

1. Multiple sclerosis, intramedullary (viral or postviral myelitis) or extramedullary (epidural abscess) infection, syringomyelia, trauma, toxins (contrast and anesthetic agents, intrathecal chemotherapy), physical agents (radiation, electrical injury), metabolic factors (chronic liver disease, vitamin B_{12} deficiency), and vascular disease (vascular malformations, infarction, hematoma).

2. The findings of abnormal signal and postcontrast enhancement within an unenlarged cord and the presence of prominent perimedullary "flow voids" suggest vascular disease, such as spinal vascular malformation.

3. The enlarged intradural vessels with "flow voids."

4. Retained contrast material within spinal cord veins, which are engorged as a result of retrograde intradural venous drainage of the fistula (located at T11), and possibly venous infarction with blood-cord barrier breakdown.

Reference

Gilbertson JR, Miller JR, Goldman MS, Marsh WR: Spinal dural arteriovenous fistulas: MR and myelographic findings. *AJNR Am J Neuroradiol* 16:2049–2057, 1995.

Cross-Reference

Neuroradiology: THE REQUISITES, pp 496–498.

Comment

The findings of cord signal abnormality and enhancement are nonspecific and may result from neoplastic, inflammatory, or vascular conditions. Cord enlargement usually favors neoplasm, although any intramedullary process that produces edema and breakdown of the blood-cord barrier may mimic neoplasm. The finding of multiple "flow voids" is the key to narrowing the differential diagnosis. Their presence favors a diagnosis of vascular malformation or vascular tumor, although collateral flow secondary to inferior vena cava occlusion or other systemic venous obstruction may be considered. The lack of flow voids within the cord makes an intramedullary arteriovenous (AV) malformation less likely than a dural AV fistula.

As for intramedullary vascular tumor, the most likely candidate is hemangioblastoma, which usually manifests findings of focal nodular enhancement and associated intramedullary cyst.

For dural AV fistulas, the approximate frequency of observation of various abnormal findings is as follows: cord hyperintensity on T2-weighted images, 90% to 100%; cord enlargement, 60% to 70%; cord enhancement (patchy or diffuse) with gadolinium, 60% to 90%; and abnormal intradural (subarachnoid) vessels, 40% to 80%. Cord enhancement results initially from spinal venous hypertension caused by the retrograde flow of blood from the fistula into the veins surrounding and within the cord. With time, venous infarction develops.

Notes

Challenge

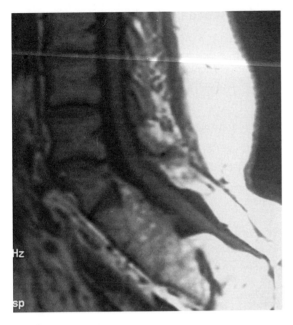 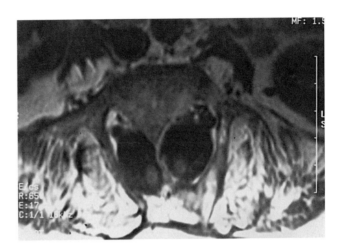

1. Name three vertebral anomalies shown by the axial T1-weighted MR image.
2. What meningeal anomaly is present?
3. Can this pathologic entity affect the filum terminale?
4. In patients with this anomaly, is the tip of the conus medullaris usually above the L2 level?

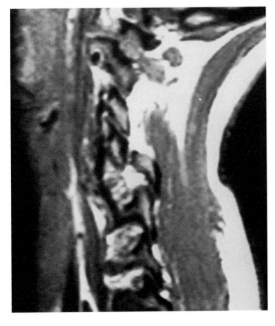 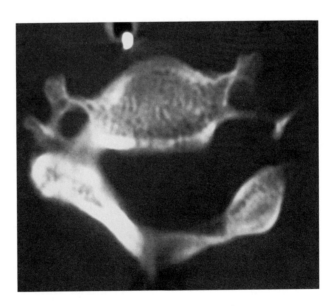

1. Is the abnormality at C5 likely to be neoplastic, infectious, congenital, or posttraumatic?
2. How does the T1-weighted parasagittal image help in making the diagnosis?
3. Is a bone scan warranted?
4. What other studies might be done if clinically indicated?

Diastematomyelia, Two Dural Sacs

1. Spina bifida, widened interpediculate distance, and midline spur or septum.

2. Two dural sacs can be seen and, consequently, two arachnoid sacs and pial membranes.

3. The midline cleft in diastematomyelia may extend through the spinal cord, conus medullaris, or filum terminale.

4. No, the tip of the conus is usually below L2 (75% of cases).

Reference

Naidich TP, Harwood-Nash DC: Diastematomyelia: Hemicord and meningeal sheath; single and double arachnoid and dural tubes. *AJNR Am J Neuroradiol* 4:633–636, 1983.

Cross-Reference

Neuroradiology: THE REQUISITES, pp 274–275.

Comment

Most of the cases of diastematomyelia with duplicated dural sacs have a fibrous or osteocartilaginous spur or septum extending through the cleft in the cord or filum. In cases with a single arachnoid and dural sac, each hemicord is surrounded by its own pial membrane, and the hemicords reportedly have no osseous or fibrous separation. Generally, the cord reunites below the cleft. These neural tube defects are best evaluated with MR imaging in conjunction with CT. In this example, the T1-weighted image demonstrates high signal intensity in the midline structure, which suggests the presence of marrow in a thick bony septum. Cortical bone, cartilage, and fibrous elements tend to have low signal intensity. Associated abnormalities that can be detected with MR imaging include tethering of the conus, myelomeningocele, hydrosyringomyelia, neurenteric cyst, and dermoid tumor.

Notes

Congenital Absence of the Pedicle

1. Congenital.

2. It demonstrates the dorsal displacement and malformation of the ipsilateral articular pillar and the enlarged intervertebral foramen without a soft tissue mass.

3. No.

4. Laboratory and imaging studies of the genitourinary system and genetic testing for neurofibromatosis.

Reference

Edwards MG, Wesolowski D, Matasar K: Imaging of the absent cervical pedicle. *Skeletal Radiol* 20:325–328, 1991.

Cross-Reference

Neuroradiology: THE REQUISITES, p 272.

Comment

Congenital absence of the pedicle is rare and typically an incidental finding. It occurs in the cervical spine less frequently than in the lumbar spine and more frequently than in the thoracic spine. It has been observed in association with genitourinary and other congenital abnormalities, as well as in patients with neurofibromatosis. This condition is distinguished from pedicle destruction by tumor or infection by the presence of fat, nerves, and vessels rather than a soft tissue mass in the widened intervertebral foramen, and by the dorsally positioned abnormal articular processes. The parasagittal T1-weighted image demonstrates an abnormal articulation at C4-5, with the inferior articular process of C4 located ventral to the C5 articular bony mass. The MR image also shows the widened C5-6 foramen with fat and neurovascular components. The different appearance of the spinous processes above and below C4-5 suggests rotation of the spine in relation to the congenital defect. These findings are confirmed on axial and reformatted sagittal CT images, which also detect sclerosis of the deformed posterior neural arch.

Notes

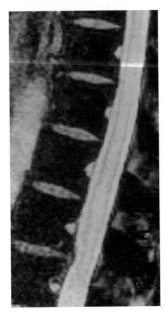
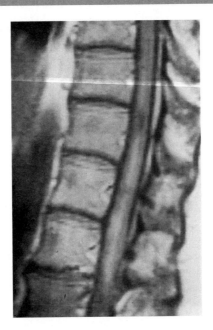

1. Do the findings on the T2-weighted and postcontrast T1-weighted MR images suggest a neoplasm?
2. What is the Foix-Alajouanine syndrome?
3. Are the MR imaging findings similar to those that have been reported for vacuolar myelopathy?
4. What MR imaging findings favor venous congestion and infarction?

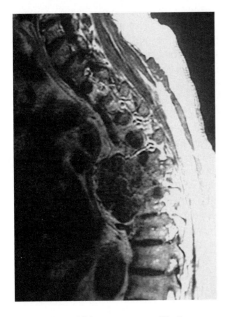
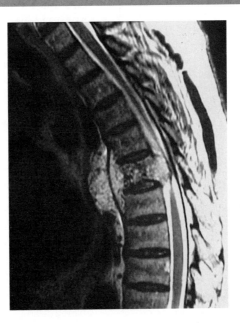

1. Is this T6 lesion more likely to represent neoplasm or infection? Why?
2. Name three neoplasms that could produce the findings on the T2-weighted sagittal image.
3. What is unusual about the mass on the T1-weighted parasagittal image?
4. How might MR imaging distinguish one type of chordoma from another?

Subacute Necrotizing Myelopathy

1. The MR imaging findings are nonspecific and in this case were due to necrotizing myelopathy.

2. Foix and Alajouanine described two patients with subacute myelopathy. The clinical syndrome consists of spastic paraparesis initially. Later, the legs become flaccid, with occasional fasciculations. A sensory deficit or paresthesia is present by the time medical attention is sought, and subsequently, bowel and bladder functions become impaired. Postmortem examination reveals extensive vascular thrombosis, spinal cord necrosis, and many abnormally dilated, tortuous, thick-walled surface vessels (veins). Many authors believe that the Foix-Alajouanine syndrome represents the end stage of chronically elevated venous pressure distal to a spinal dural arteriovenous fistula. Some authors have stressed that this syndrome is not synonymous with subacute necrotizing myelopathy, which encompasses a broader spectrum of disease.

3. Enhancement on postcontrast T1-weighted images, as shown here, is atypical for vacuolar myelopathy in AIDS.

4. Diffuse cord signal abnormalities in association with enlargement and tortuosity of vessels (veins) on the cord surface. The finding of enlarged perimedullary and not intramedullary vessels would favor venous congestion and infarction in the cord.

References

Criscuolo GR, Oldfield EH, Doppman JL: Reversible acute and subacute myelopathy in patients with dural arteriovenous fistulas. Foix-Alajouanine syndrome revisited. *J Neurosurg* 70:354–359, 1989.

Mirich DR, Kucharczyk W, Keller MA, Deck J: Subacute necrotizing myelopathy: MR imaging in four pathologically proved cases. *AJNR Am J Neuroradiol* 12:1077–1083, 1991.

Cross-Reference

Neuroradiology: THE REQUISITES, p 498.

Comment

Subacute necrotizing myelopathy is a clinicopathologic entity characterized by progressive ascending sensory and motor deficits and loss of sphincter control that develop rapidly and often end with complete quadriplegia and intercostal paralysis. Pathologic examination reveals necrosis with little or no inflammation. Both gray and white matter are affected, and the thoracolumbar region is preferentially involved. Spinal cord arteries are normal. This entity may result from a variety of conditions, including systemic infections (mumps, rubeola, mononucleosis), toxic agents (iodochlorhydroxyquin intoxication), malignancies with paraneoplastic syndrome (leukemia), and vascular disease (thrombophlebitis, spinal dural fistula). The cord may be normal in size or enlarged, with diffuse T2 hyperintensity and postcontrast enhancement. The differential diagnosis includes infectious myelitis, astrocytoma, and arterial infarction.

Chordoma, Thoracic

1. Neoplasm, because the disk spaces and end-plates are relatively spared.

2. The neoplastic lesions that are most likely to show paraspinal, intraosseous, and epidural involvement are metastases (breast, lung primaries), lymphoma, and plasmacytoma.

3. The signal intensity is very low and appears similar to that of CSF and much lower than that of the posterior paraspinous muscles.

4. Some evidence indicates that chondroid chordomas, which have abundant cartilage-like tissue, are hypointense in comparison with typical chordomas on T2-weighted images. The amount of the cartilage-like component in chondroid chordomas, though, is variable and often minimal, so the hyperintense cystic/mucinous features observed with typical chordomas frequently predominate.

Reference

Murphy JM, Wallis F, Toland J, Toner M, Wilson GF: CT and MRI appearances of a thoracic chordoma. *Eur Radiol* 8:1677–1679, 1998.

Cross-Reference

Neuroradiology: THE REQUISITES, p 494.

Comment

Chordomas account for less than 5% of primary malignant bone tumors. They arise from intraosseous notochordal remnants and are slow growing and lobulated. Two types are distinguished histopathologically: typical chordomas, which have a watery, gelatinous matrix, and chondroid chordomas, in which this matrix is replaced by cartilaginous foci. Because of these characteristics, chordomas may have relatively low signal intensity in comparison to muscle on T1-weighted images, as in this case. Signal intensity is usually inhomogeneous, however, because a combination of cystic and solid components frequently exists. Lesions demonstrating high signal intensity on T1-weighted images have been reported. On T2-weighted images, inhomogeneous signal intensity is also observed, with some regions of the tumor equaling or exceeding the intensity of CSF. In a recent report of a thoracic chordoma, the authors observed that septa of low signal intensity radiated throughout the predominantly high-signal-intensity mass on T2-weighted images—a feature that may help in differentiating chordomas from the more common paraspinal/spinal masses. In order of decreasing frequency, the location of chordoma is reported to be sacrococcygeal (50%–60%), skull base (25%–35%), and cervicothoracolumbar vertebral bodies (approximately 15%).

The very low signal intensity of the mass on T1-weighted images would be unusual for highly cellular tumors such as lymphoma and plasmacytoma, but it could be consistent with osteoblastic metastases. Calcification occurs in 30% to 70% of chordomas, and thus CT may be helpful in the differential diagnosis. Postcontrast enhancement of chordomas is variable. A few cases of completely extradural, extraosseous vertebral chordomas have been reported.

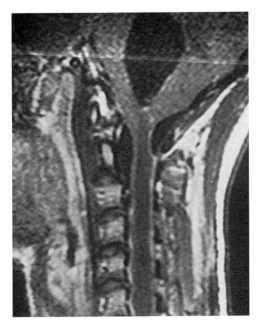
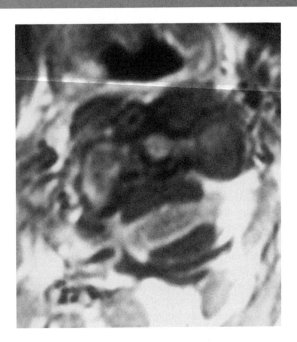

1. Do the findings on these *postcontrast* images suggest a congenital or an acquired disorder?

2. What imaging study would you recommend next?

3. How can you rule in or rule out CNS infection or tumor?

4. Are the signal changes in the cord consistent with hydromyelia, syringomyelia, or myelomalacia?

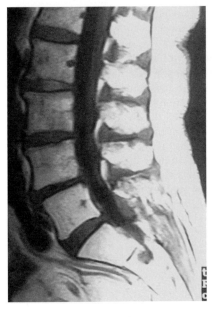
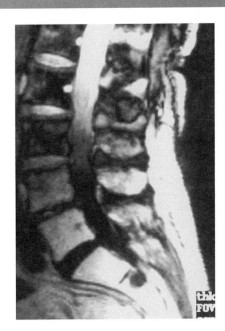

1. In this patient with a recurrent pelvic sarcoma, which spinal level(s) is (are) involved based on the T1-weighted (left) and fat-suppressed, fast-spin-echo (FSE), proton-density-weighted (right) images?

2. How do you explain the high signal intensity within the L5 and S1 vertebral bodies on both images?

3. What additional imaging should be done in this patient?

4. List three methods of fat suppression.

Chronic Coccidioidal Meningitis With Syringomyelia*

1. Acquired. The tonsils are not frankly ectopic, as would be expected for Chiari I or II malformations, but rather are compressed by extraaxial fluid collections at the foramen magnum.

2. MR imaging or CT of the brain to determine the pattern and severity of ventricular dilatation.

3. Usually by obtaining CSF for analysis, which may be done at the time of ventriculostomy placement. Lumbar puncture is contraindicated because of the potential for tonsillar herniation.

4. Syringomyelia. The cord is diffusely enlarged and homogeneously hypointense centrally, consistent with a cyst rather than myelomalacia. The fluid in the cyst is hyperintense to CSF, as occurs with purulent or proteinaceous fluid. In hydromyelia the signal characteristics and composition of the fluid are the same as CSF. The final diagnosis depends on the lining of the cyst or cavity—ependymal lining in hydromyelia and glial lining in syringomyelia.

References

Gupta RK, Gupta S, Kumar S, Kohli A, Misra UK, Gujral RB: Central nervous system tuberculosis: MRI. *Neuroradiology* 36:93–96, 1994.

Madsen PW III, Bowen BC: Spinal cord disease. In: Kelley RE, Ed: *Functional Neuroimaging.* Armonk, NY, Futura, 1994, pp 415–447.

Cross-Reference

Neuroradiology: THE REQUISITES, pp 478–480, 484–485.

Comment

The important findings in this case are the enlarged fourth ventricle, absence of vermian interfolial folds, extraaxial CSF-equivalent fluid collections and hyperintensity (enhancement) of the cord surface at the craniocervical junction, and syringomyelia. The constellation of findings suggests a chronic infection causing thickened leptomeninges (pachymeningitis). Involvement of the basal cisterns and spinal subarachnoid space results in (1) basal meningitis, which is responsible for the hydrocephalus, and (2) spinal arachnoiditis, which is responsible for the syringomyelia, probable subarachnoid cysts, and scattered leptomeningeal enhancement. Abnormal flow of CSF at the foramen magnum contributes to the development of syringomyelia. The syrinx does not communicate with the fourth ventricle, as evidenced here by the difference in signal intensity between the fourth ventricle and the syrinx, which extends to the obex. Infections most likely to elicit a host granulomatous inflammatory response and produce the above findings are tuberculosis (*Mycobacterium tuberculosis*), coccidioidomycosis (*Coccidioides immitis*), and cysticercosis (*Taenia solium*).

*Sagittal image from Madsen PW III, Bowen BC: Spinal cord disease. In: Kelley RE, Ed: *Functional Neuroimaging.* Armonk, NY, Futura, 1994.

Inhomogeneous Fat Suppression

1. A lytic lesion is located at S2.

2. The high signal intensity is due to fatty marrow. It is present on the proton-density-weighted FSE image because of a lack of fat saturation.

3. The fat saturation pulse sequence should be repeated after reshimming of the magnetic field to achieve more homogeneous fat suppression. Alternatively, a short tau inversion recovery (STIR) image should be obtained.

4. Chemical shift fat saturation, STIR, and Dixon (subtraction of in-phase and out-of-phase image data yielding either "water" or "fat" images) methods.

References

Simon JH, Rubinstein D: Contrast-enhanced fat-suppression neuroimaging. *Neuroimaging Clin N Am* 4:153–173, 1994.

Tien RD, Olson EM, Zee CS: Diseases of the lumbar spine: Findings on fat-suppression MR imaging. *AJR Am J Roentgenol* 159:95–99, 1992.

Cross-Reference

Neuroradiology: THE REQUISITES, pp 453–455.

Comment

The method of fat suppression used in the proton-density-weighted FSE image is chemical shift fat saturation. Ideally, in this method a radiofrequency (RF) pulse of narrow bandwidth saturates the signal from fat protons before data acquisition; however, if the magnetic field is not homogeneous because of inadequate or ineffective shimming, the fat resonance in some areas may occur at a frequency outside the saturation pulse bandwidth. In this case, no suppression of fat signal occurs in the corresponding parts of the image. If the field inhomogeneity is such that the water proton resonance in some areas falls within the saturation pulse bandwidth, the water signal will be saturated in those parts of the image. This scenario is what has occurred for the FSE acquisition. Below the level of L3–4, saturation of the water signal and not the fat signal by the RF pulse results in dark CSF and bright vertebrae. Above L3–4, the RF pulse saturates the fat signal as expected, and dark vertebrae and relatively bright CSF are produced. When the chemical shift saturation method produces image artifacts as a result of field inhomogeneity, more uniform fat suppression can generally be obtained by using the STIR method with a long recovery time (TR) to generate images with proton density or T2 weighting.

Notes

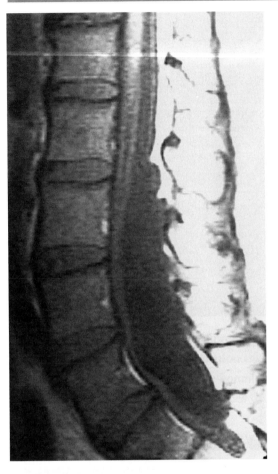
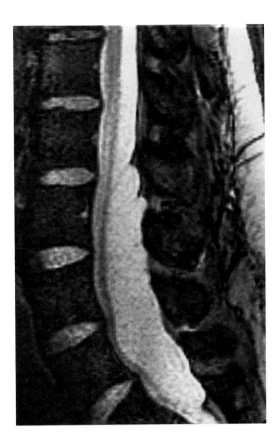
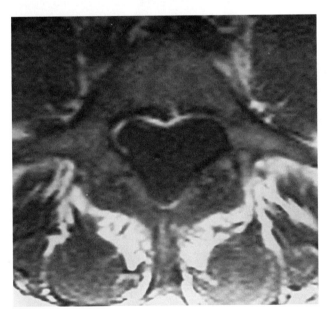

1. Why is this not a classic meningocele?

2. Why is this unlikely to be arachnoiditis?

3. Would this be classified as a type II meningeal cyst?

4. This patient was referred for MR imaging because of bilateral leg edema and weakness. Her history includes recurrent conjunctivitis. You want to interview this patient. Why?

Radiation-Induced Malignant Fibrous Histiocytoma

1. Ependymoma.

2. Hyperintense vertebrae, abnormal cord signal intensity and size, and secondary malignancies.

3. Secondary.

4. Osteosarcoma, fibrosarcoma, and spindle cell sarcoma.

Reference

Nadeem SQ, Feun LG, Bruce-Gregorios JH, Green B: Post radiation sarcoma (malignant fibrous histiocytoma) of the cervical spine following ependymoma (a case report). *J Neurooncol* 11:263-268, 1991.

Cross-Reference

Neuroradiology: THE REQUISITES, p 482.

Comment

In terms of the differential diagnosis, the most important finding on the precontrast and postcontrast T1-weighted images is the diffuse hyperintensity involving the cervical vertebrae. This finding represents the conversion of normal bone marrow to fatty marrow as a result of spinal irradiation. In addition to radiation therapy, an extensive laminectomy (C1-7) has been performed. The cord demonstrates abnormal enhancement, without enlargement, at C4 and C5. The most plausible explanation for these findings is that the patient has been treated for an intramedullary neoplasm. Although less common than ependymoma, astrocytoma tends to involve the cervicothoracic region and would be treated by radiation rather than total or subtotal resection. The cord enhancement may represent residual intramedullary tumor, radiation myelitis, or possibly cord invasion from the posterior, peripherally enhancing mass. The mass, however, appears predominantly extradural and distinct from the intramedullary lesion. Although the differential diagnosis includes lymphoma, metastatic disease, or invasive primary bone malignancy, the radiation changes should prompt a diagnosis of radiation-induced malignancy. The majority of postradiation malignancies are sarcomas. CNS tumors that have developed after radiation therapy (in some cases combined with chemotherapy) include meningiomas and astrocytomas. Thus, the differential diagnosis might include treated extradural malignancy with postradiation cervical astrocytoma.

Ten years before this MR imaging study, the patient had partial resection and irradiation for a "grade II astrocytoma," which subsequently proved to be an "ependymoma with some astrocytic components" rather than a low-grade astrocytoma. Subtotal resection of the posterior mass shown here revealed malignant fibrous histiocytoma (MFH). Postradiation MFH is very rare.

Notes

Hodgkin's Lymphoma, Postchemotherapy

1. Fat replacement of bone marrow.

2. Chemical shift, fat saturation imaging.

3. Chemotherapy.

4. Six weeks.

References

Lien HH, Holte H: Fat replacement of Hodgkin disease of bone marrow after chemotherapy: Report of three cases. *Skeletal Radiol* 25:671-674, 1996.

Stevens SK, Moore SG, Kaplan ID: Early and late bone-marrow changes after irradiation: MR evaluation. *AJR Am J Roentgenol* 154:745-750, 1990.

Cross-Reference

Neuroradiology: THE REQUISITES, pp 481-482.

Comment

The right parasagittal image demonstrates better than does the axial image the diffusely increased signal intensity within the T8 vertebra. The axial image shows right epidural, foraminal, and paraspinal soft tissue tumor. Imaging was performed 12 weeks after chemotherapy for Hodgkin's disease. Either chemotherapy alone or radiation therapy alone could produce the signal characteristics of fat replacement shown here. Radiation therapy, however, usually produces changes in more than one vertebra because of the size of the treatment field. Patients treated with spinal irradiation usually manifest increased signal on T1-weighted images after a time interval of 6 weeks or more. For chemotherapy to produce the signal intensity shown here, the malignant tumor must first have destroyed the hematopoietic and stromal supportive tissue in the vertebra. Then chemotherapy must have eradicated the tumor, thereby allowing fat to repopulate the marrow space. The differential diagnosis for the MR imaging findings includes asymptomatic vertebral hemangioma; however, vertebral hemangiomas that are aggressive and extend beyond the vertebral margins tend to be hypointense on T1-weighted images because of their predominantly angiomatous stroma.

While STIR (short tau inversion recovery) sequences are useful to eliminate signal from fat, they may also suppress the signal from hemorrhage or other substances with a short T1 relaxation time. Chemical shift–selective, fat saturation pulses, on the other hand, saturate the signal from resonances in the 1- to 2-ppm range (lipid region) of the proton spectrum and would not be expected to suppress the signal from hemorrhage. Thus, elimination of high signal in the affected vertebra by chemical shift fat saturation provides more conclusive evidence that the signal abnormality is due to fat replacement.

Notes

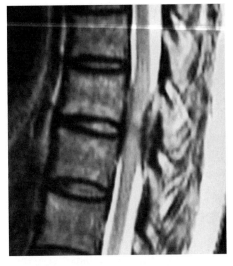
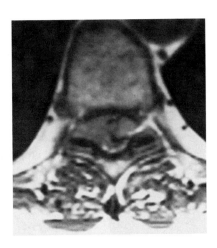
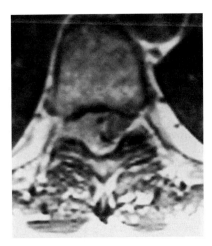

1. Is the location of this T8-9 lesion primarily intramedullary, extramedullary intradural, or extradural?

2. What additional imaging study would help narrow the differential diagnosis?

3. What spinal tumor behaves more aggressively when it is extradural than when it is intradural?

4. How would the finding of a widened neural foramen affect your differential diagnosis?

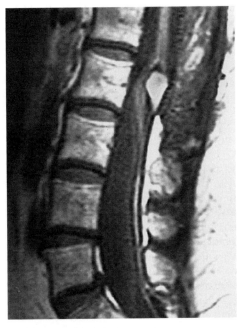
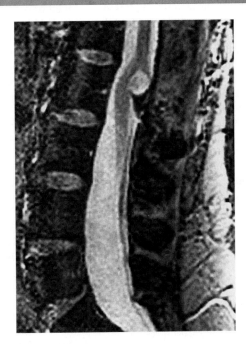

1. In these T1- and T2*-weighted sagittal images, is this lesion more likely acquired or congenital?

2. Name three types of lesions that commonly have intramedullary and extramedullary components.

3. What lumbosacral dysraphic defect may be present?

4. What intracranial finding may aid in the diagnosis of this lesion?

Pantopaque Mimicking Intradural Lipoma

1. The findings on intraoperative ultrasound are those of a cystic, rather than solid, mass.

2. Iophendylate (trade names Pantopaque and Myodil). Iothalamate is an intravascular contrast agent.

3. Arachnoiditis.

4. Arachnoiditis is reportedly more likely to occur if iophendylate is mixed with blood during a traumatic spinal tap or spinal surgery.

Reference

Hughes DG, Isherwood I: How frequent is chronic lumbar arachnoiditis following intrathecal Myodil? *Br J Radiol* 65:758–760, 1992.

Cross-Reference

Neuroradiology: THE REQUISITES, p 472.

Comment

Iophendylate (Pantopaque) was the most commonly used oil-based contrast agent for myelography in the United States before 1980. Although oil based, it is heavier than water and seeks a dependent location within the CSF-containing subarachnoid space. Because of its short T1 relaxation time, it is hyperintense on T1-weighted images and thus mimics lipoma or subacute hemorrhage. In some cases, the hydrophobic droplets of Pantopaque will migrate to different locations along the spinal axis upon repositioning of the patient. In this case, intraoperative ultrasound demonstrates two regions with similar acoustic impedance separated by a thin, mildly echogenic border. The regions are uniformly hypoechoic, and both demonstrate marked "through transmission," consistent with cystic properties—one region represents the lumbar subarachnoid space, whereas the other represents the Pantopaque "droplet."

Although the procedure for iophendylate studies was to remove all the oil after the myelogram, residual contrast could be difficult to retrieve. In the radiology literature are reports that chronic exposure to the agent, apparently exacerbated by the presence of blood initially, can result in lumbar arachnoiditis. Some investigators, however, have presented evidence that iophendylate (introduced by ventriculostomy or cisternal puncture) rarely produces lumbar arachnoiditis. In the sagittal MR image, no cauda equina nerve roots are visible. This appearance results from arachnoiditis with adhesions that draw the roots to the margin of the thecal sac ("empty sac" sign).

Notes

Hemangioendothelioma

1. Complete vertebral rather than hemivertebral stain, nonhomogeneous stain extending outside the confines of the bone, hypervascularity, and early-draining vessel caudally.

2. Thyroid carcinoma and renal cell carcinoma.

3. Supreme intercostal branch of the right subclavian artery.

4. Hyperintensity on T1-weighted images due to fatty overgrowth.

Reference

Murphey MD, Fairbairn KJ, Parman LM, Baxter KG, Parsa MB, Smith WS: From the archives of the AFIP. Musculoskeletal angiomatous lesions: Radiologic-pathologic correlation. *Radiographics* 15:893–917, 1995.

Cross-Reference

Neuroradiology: THE REQUISITES, pp 493–494.

Comment

The frontal radiograph demonstrates lytic changes within the T2 vertebral body, without loss of height, and the right subclavian arteriogram reveals a hypervascular mass with findings described in answer 1 above. While benign hemangiomas may have similar findings, the differential diagnosis must include more aggressive vascular tumors, primarily hemangioendothelioma, hemangiopericytoma, and angiosarcoma. The first two are of intermediate aggressiveness and may be benign or malignant, whereas the third is a very aggressive, malignant neoplasm. When any one of the three neoplasms involves the spine, the most common clinical findings are myelopathy from cord compression and pain caused by extradural extension of tumor.

The three neoplasms cannot be differentiated radiologically. When compared with hemangioma, they are more likely to cause marked osseous expansion, penetration of the cortex, and an associated soft tissue mass. They are frequently multifocal with intervening normal bone. Angiographically, hemangiopericytoma is more likely than the others to show a vascular pedicle entering the mass. On MR imaging, signal changes induced by vascular channels (flow voids caused by high flow or increased T2 signal associated with slow flow) are evident. The fatty overgrowth associated with most hemangiomas is absent. Hemangioendothelioma arises from vascular endothelial cells and has several histologic subtypes (spindle cell, epithelioid, and kaposiform). Osseous lesions are more common in young men. Associated angiomatous syndromes include Maffucci's, Klippel-Trenaunay-Weber, and Kasabach-Merritt.

Notes

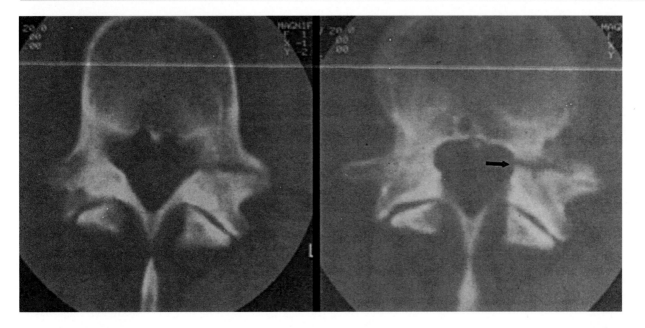

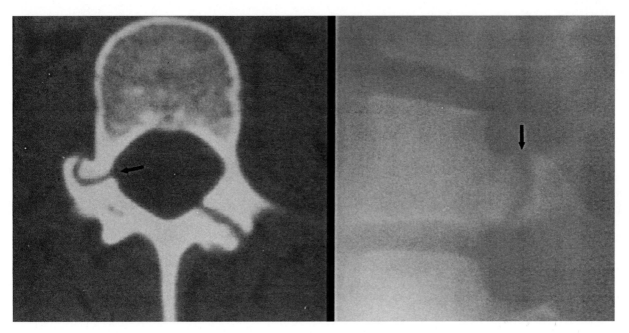

1. You are shown adjacent CT images from one patient and a CT image plus a lateral radiograph from a second patient. What is the name of the bony defect (*arrow*) that these patients have in common?

2. Why is this defect not spondylolysis?

3. The second patient has bilateral bony defects. Is the defect involving the left side of the neural arch typically seen in association with the right-sided defect?

4. Why is the defect (*arrow*) not persistent neurocentral synchondrosis?

Retrosomatic Cleft

1. Retrosomatic cleft.

2. The bony defect in spondylolysis occurs posterior to the transverse process.

3. No. The left-sided defect is a retroisthmic cleft. A retrosomatic cleft has been shown to be associated with contralateral spondylolysis (pars defect), not a retroisthmic cleft.

4. Persistent neurocentral synchondrosis involves the posterolateral aspect of the vertebral body, not the pedicle (as shown here).

References

Johansen JG, McCarty DJ, Haughton VM: Retrosomatic clefts: Computed tomographic appearance. *Radiology* 148:447–448, 1983.
Osborn RE, el-Khoury GY, Lehmann TR: Retrosomatic cleft: A radiographic study. *Spine* 12:950–952, 1987.

Cross-Reference

Neuroradiology: THE REQUISITES, pp 274, 449–451, 459.

Comment

The CT images and the lateral radiograph demonstrate a pedicular defect (*arrows*) that has relatively smooth margins and no definite evidence of healing. Neither patient gave a history of trauma, thus supporting a diagnosis of retrosomatic cleft. This rare congenital defect involves the pedicle and probably results from anomalous ossification centers. It is most commonly found in women older than 30 years. Its location anterior to the transverse process differentiates it from spondylolysis, retroisthmic cleft, and spina bifida (all located posterior to the transverse process). Its pedicular location differentiates it from persistent neurocentral synchondrosis, which represents a failure of fusion of the three vertebral body ossification centers. Its coronal orientation, short length, and usual smooth margins differentiate it from pedicular hypoplasia or aplasia. Retrosomatic cleft is believed to be congenital rather than posttraumatic, and an article describing cartilage obtained from the cleft supports this theory. Hypertrophic changes adjacent to the cleft may be present. It has been suggested that retrosomatic clefts are of no clinical significance unless they lead to disk degeneration.

Notes

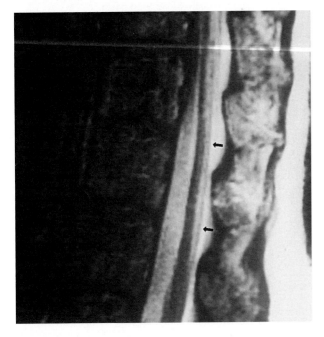
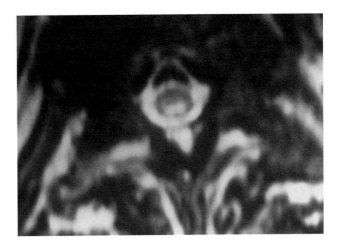

1. Name four conditions that may produce the intramedullary hyperintensity shown on the T2-weighted images.

2. What metabolic disease is usually responsible for this finding?

3. What intraoperative treatment may contribute to this finding?

4. What patient population has shown an increased prevalence of this disease?

Subacute Combined Degeneration

1. Multiple sclerosis, wallerian degeneration (e.g., posttraumatic), arterial ischemia or infarction, and metabolic disease. Other possibilities include postinfectious myelitis and radiation myelitis.

2. Vitamin B_{12} deficiency.

3. Nitrous oxide anesthesia during surgery.

4. HIV-positive patients, especially those with AIDS.

References

Timms SR, Cure JK, Kurent JE: Subacute combined degeneration of the spinal cord: MR findings. *AJNR Am J Neuroradiol* 14:1224–1227, 1993.

Yamada K, Shrier DA, Tanaka H, Numaguchi Y: A case of subacute combined degeneration: MRI findings. *Neuroradiology* 40:398–400, 1998.

Cross-Reference

Neuroradiology: THE REQUISITES, p 480.

Comment

Bilaterally symmetric, increased signal intensity is seen in the posterior columns (*arrows*) of the thoracic cord on the T2-weighted images, without cord enlargement (the hypointensities anteriorly within the canal are "flow voids"). The abnormal cord signal represents subacute combined degeneration (SCD), which is the manifestation of vitamin B_{12} deficiency in the spinal cord. Often, the signal abnormality appears as an upside-down V. This configuration reflects greater involvement of the lateral than the medial portions of the dorsal columns and would correspond to relative sparing of proprioceptive sensation in the lower extremities clinically. Histopathologic studies demonstrate degeneration of myelin sheaths and axonal loss in the posterior *and lateral* columns. Despite histologic evidence of lateral column lesions and clinical evidence of lateral corticospinal tract involvement in some reported cases, hyperintense MR signal has been observed primarily in the posterior columns, with only occasional MR imaging evidence of posterior and lateral column involvement.

Two cases of SCD with posterior column hyperintensity on T2-weighted images and postcontrast MR imaging have been reported. In the first case, posterior column enhancement without cord enlargement was seen, whereas in the second case, cord enlargement without posterior column enhancement was noted.

Vitamin B_{12} (cyanocobalamin) deficiency may result from insufficient ingestion or impaired intestinal absorption (e.g., lack of intrinsic factor, total or partial gastrectomy, celiac disease, Crohn's disease, and chronic pancreatic insufficiency) of vitamin B_{12}. The most common cause of vitamin B_{12} deficiency in the United States is pernicious anemia, which results from an insufficiency of intrinsic factor, a binding protein secreted by gastric parietal cells. An underlying autoimmune disorder is believed to be responsible since most patients have circulating antibodies to parietal cells or lymphocytic infiltration of gastric mucosa. In recent years, an increasing prevalence of vitamin B_{12} deficiency has been reported in HIV-positive patients, especially those with AIDS.

In patients with borderline vitamin B_{12} serum levels, SCD may be promoted by the administration of nitrous oxide anesthesia during surgery (or by nitrous oxide abuse). Nitrous oxide enhances the oxidation and hence inactivation of vitamin B_{12}.

Notes

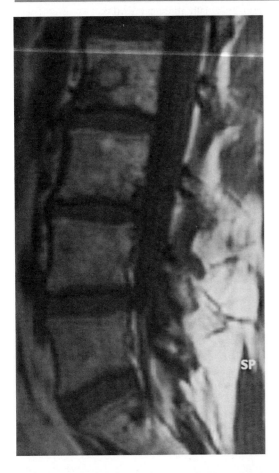

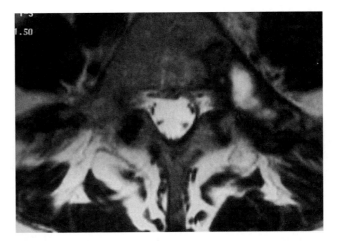

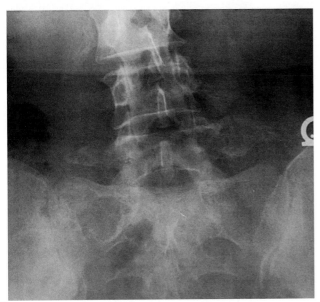

1. This 43-year-old woman has a history of chronic back pain and hyperthyroidism. Based on the MR imaging and radiographic findings, what additional clinical information would you like to have to make the diagnosis?

2. Is dural ectasia a feature of this disease?

3. List four nonmalignant lesions that may produce the findings at L5.

4. Give five examples of primary tumors that have osteoblastic metastases.

Polyostotic Fibrous Dysplasia

1. Information regarding whether the patient has abnormal skin pigmentation. The imaging findings are compatible with polyostotic fibrous dysplasia, and the history of an endocrine disorder raises the possibility of McCune-Albright syndrome. The syndrome also includes the presence of pigmented areas, referred to as café au lait spots, with a jagged ("coast of Maine") outline.

2. Dural ectasia is a feature of neurofibromatosis type 1, not fibrous dysplasia.

3. Osteoblastoma, giant cell tumor, nonossifying fibroma, and fibrous dysplasia.

4. Prostate, breast, carcinoid, ovarian, and transitional cell carcinoma. Lymphoma may also appear as an osteoblastic lesion.

References

Hoffman KL, Bergman AG, Kohler S: Polyostotic fibrous dysplasia with severe pathologic compression fracture of L2. *Skeletal Radiol* 24:160–162, 1995.

Przybylski GJ, Pollack IF, Ward WT: Monostotic fibrous dysplasia of the thoracic spine. A case report. *Spine* 21:860–865, 1996.

Cross-Reference

Neuroradiology: THE REQUISITES, pp 491–495.

Comment

The sagittal T1-weighted image of this patient with McCune-Albright syndrome shows a lesion in the body of L2 that has an isointense center and hypointense rim. Focal hypointense areas are evident near the inferior end-plates of L2 and L3 and the body of S1. On the axial T2-weighted image, a lesion involving the left pedicle and transverse process of L5 has a hyperintense center and extensive hypointense periphery. The plain radiograph reveals expansile, trabeculated lesions of the left L5 and L4 transverse processes, a relatively lucent left L5 pedicle in comparison with the normal right L5 pedicle, and increased density on the right side of L3. In addition, the S1 right sacral ala has a radiolucent area. The MR imaging findings are representative of fibrous dysplasia, in which signal intensity is variable and depends on the relative amounts of fibrous, cartilaginous, and sometimes, hemorrhagic components. Typically, the lesions are of intermediate to low signal intensity on T1-weighted images. On T2-weighted images, fibrous regions have low signal intensity, whereas predominantly cartilaginous regions have high signal intensity.

In general, fibrous dysplasia is more commonly monostotic (85%) than polyostotic (15%). In polyostotic disease, localized skin pigmentation (café au lait spots) is present in about one third of patients. Associated endocrine manifestations include hyperthyroidism, acromegaly, Cushing's syndrome, and sexual precocity. The association of polyostotic involvement with cutaneous and endocrine manifestations is termed the McCune-Albright syndrome. It occurs in up to 50% of females with polyostotic disease. Malignant transformation of fibrous dysplasia to sarcoma is very uncommon (0.5%).

In the spine, fibrous dysplasia is more commonly polyostotic than monostotic. The incidence of spinal involvement in polyostotic disease ranges from 7% in the cervical spine to 14% in the lumbar spine. Monostotic fibrous dysplasia of the spine is exceedingly rare, but case reports (fewer than 30) of solitary cervical, thoracic, and lumbar lesions have appeared in the literature. In the majority of cases of fibrous dysplasia of the spine, the lesions are asymptomatic and require no treatment. Many patients do have spinal pain, and a few examples of pathologic compression fractures, with or without trauma, have been reported.

Notes

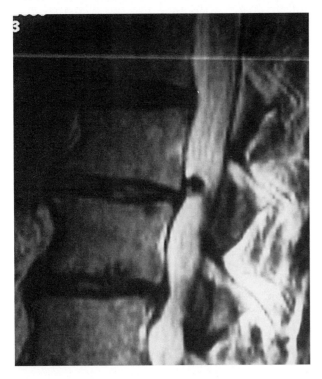

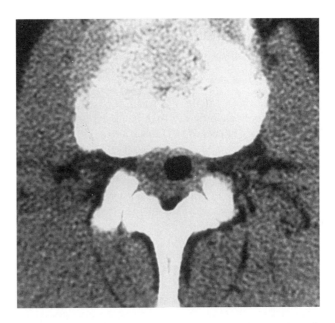

1. What is the composition of the focal low-intensity and low-density region within the spinal canal at L1-2 in this 66-year-old man with chronic, multilevel degenerative disk disease?

2. Name three types of lesions that may contain such a region.

3. Which is more sensitive in detecting intradiskal gas collections—spin-echo or gradient-echo MR imaging?

4. Which motion is said to promote the appearance or enlargement of a "vacuum phenomenon" in the intervertebral disk space—flexion or extension of the spine?

Intraspinal Gas Collection

1. Gas collection, predominantly nitrogen.

2. Disk herniation, synovial cyst, and free gas in the epidural space.

3. Gradient-echo MR imaging.

4. Extension.

Reference

Pierpaolo L, Luciano M, Fabrizio P, Paolo M: Gas-containing lumbar disc herniation. A case report and review of the literature. *Spine* 18:2533–2536, 1993.

Cross-Reference

Neuroradiology: THE REQUISITES, pp 460, 466–467.

Comment

The left parasagittal T2-weighted image shows focal low signal intensity posterior and superior to the L1-2 disk space. This feature could represent gas, hemorrhage, calcification, or vascular flow void. The hyperintense superior rim of the lesion represents a susceptibility artifact. On the CT image, the lesion is markedly hypodense, consistent with a gas collection. While the gas collection contacts the disk space, the presence or absence of a thin rim of "soft" disk material surrounding the gas cannot be determined. No "vacuum phenomenon" is present within the L1-2 disk space.

It is generally accepted that a gas collection like the one shown here is pathognomonic of disk herniation, either extradural or, less commonly, intradural. Some authors, however, have proposed several etiologies, including (1) free gas in the epidural space (occurs only at the level of an intervertebral disk space with a vacuum phenomenon), (2) "gas bubbles" with a reactive peripheral fibrous capsule (the capsule, however, may merely represent an old disk protrusion in which the wall has become thinned because of progressive degeneration accompanied by enlargement of the gas collection), and (3) herniation of the nucleus pulposus of an intervertebral disk that already has a vacuum phenomenon.

The vacuum phenomenon within an intervertebral space represents the accumulation of gas in preexisting diskal fissures or cavities in response to decreased intradiskal pressure caused by external forces applied to the spine or by hyperextension of the spine. Intervertebral gas collections reportedly increase with extension and decrease with flexion of the spine. They are composed of nitrogen (90%–92%) combined primarily with oxygen and carbon dioxide.

Intraspinal gas collections that appear to be causing nerve root compression have been "treated" by percutaneous aspiration with an 18-gauge spinal needle. Preliminary results indicate that symptoms can be alleviated for at least several months.

Notes

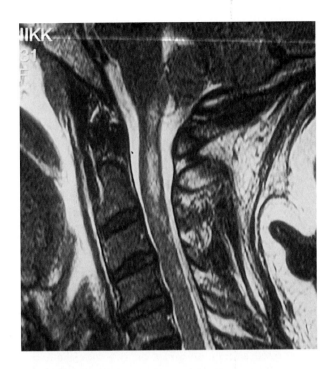

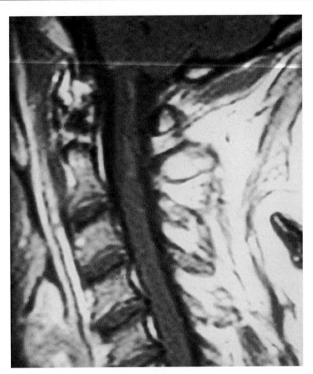

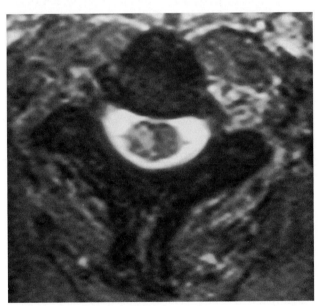

1. What spinal cord syndrome is this patient likely to have?

2. What syndrome is commonly associated with demyelinating lesions?

3. What syndrome is often seen with hyperextension injuries in the neck?

4. List three spinal cord syndromes produced by vascular insults. Which is most common?

Unilateral Cord Infarction, Cervical

1. Brown-Séquard, or cord hemisection, syndrome consisting of ipsilateral spastic paresis, contralateral loss of pain/temperature sensation below the level of the lesion, and ipsilateral loss of proprioceptive sensation. In this case, relative sparing of ipsilateral proprioceptive sensation has resulted in a partial Brown-Séquard syndrome.

2. Posterior cord syndrome: pain and paresthesias are present and are out of proportion to motor impairment in the affected segments.

3. Central cord syndrome.

4. Anterior cord syndrome (anterior spinal artery occlusion), which is the most common; posterior cord syndrome (posterior spinal artery occlusion); and partial Brown-Séquard syndrome (anterior or posterior spinal artery occlusion).

References

Bergqvist CA, Goldberg HI, Thorarensen O, Bird SJ: Posterior cervical spinal cord infarction following vertebral artery dissection. *Neurology* 48:1112–1115, 1997.

de la Sayette V, Leproux F, Letellier P: Cervical cord and dorsal medullary infarction presenting with retro-orbital pain. *Neurology* 53:632–634, 1999.

Cross-Reference

Neuroradiology: THE REQUISITES, pp 495–496.

Comment

The distal right vertebral artery in this 43-year-old woman was embolized to control the loss of blood from a large posterior inferior communicating artery aneurysm that had ruptured during attempted embolization with Guglielmi detachable coils (GDC). Subsequently, weakness developed on the right side of the patient's body (upper and lower extremities), and loss of pain/temperature sense developed on the left side, with relative sparing of vibratory and joint position sense. The MR imaging study was obtained 5 days after embolization and shows hyperintensity on the right side of the cord at C1-2 on the T2-weighted sagittal and T2*-weighted axial (C2 level) images. The axial image demonstrates the abrupt margin of the lesion at the midline of the cord and some sparing of the white matter of the posterior and lateral columns. Minimal patchy, elongated enhancement is observed on the postcontrast T1-weighted image, without obvious cord enlargement. The findings are not typical for demyelinating disease, which should exhibit predominantly peripheral (white matter) rather than central (gray matter) involvement, or for intramedullary primary tumor (astrocytoma, ependymoma), which usually causes cord enlargement, more prominent enhancement than shown here, and cyst formation (25%–50% of cases approximately).

The anterior spinal artery supplies the anterior two thirds of the cord parenchyma. It is derived from paired longitudinal vessels that fuse over most of their length by the second embryonic month. Unfused portions appear as duplications or fenestrations, most often seen in the cervical region. In the upper cervical spine, anterior medullary (or radiculomedullary) arteries from the vertebral arteries supply the anterior spinal artery. A plausible explanation for the findings in this case is that the patient has a duplicated cervical segment of the anterior spinal artery and that this segment is supplied by radiculomedullary branches of the right vertebral artery. Occlusion of the right vertebral artery caused an abrupt loss of blood to the right limb of the anterior spinal artery and ultimately resulted in a unilateral infarct and symptoms of a partial Brown-Séquard syndrome. Unilateral cervical cord infarctions can also occur with a single anterior spinal artery. The occluded vessel (or vessels) in this case is a sulcal artery that originates from the anterior spinal artery in the anterior median fissure and courses centrally and then to the right or left to supply central gray matter. Because adjacent sulcal arteries alternate their supply to the right and left sides of the cord (right, then left, then right for successive sulcal arteries) and because the single anterior spinal artery is supplied by both vertebral arteries, it is rare to have a unilateral infarct resulting from occlusion of a single vertebral artery.

The paired posterior spinal arteries supply the posterior third of the cord parenchyma, including the posterior columns, posterior horns, and posterolateral portion of the lateral columns. In the upper cervical spine these arteries are supplied by posterior medullary (or radiculopial) arteries, which originate primarily from the vertebral arteries. Because the posterior spinal arteries are part of the rich anastomotic pial network on the cord surface, it is unusual to have a posterior cord infarct. Examples of a single posterior medullary artery supplying both posterior spinal arteries have been reported, however, and in one case (Berggvist and colleagues), right vertebral artery dissection resulted in bilateral posterior spinal artery territory infarction and a posterior cord syndrome.

Notes

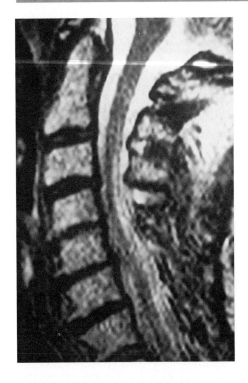

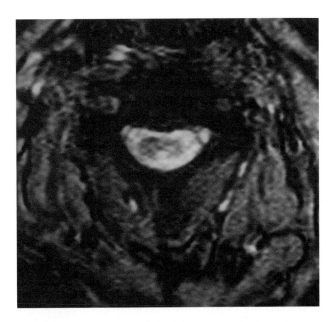

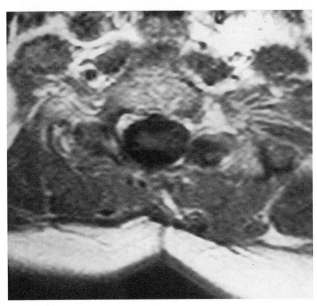

1. Name two metabolic diseases that may produce the MR imaging findings in the spinal cord shown on the T2-weighted sagittal and the T2*-weighted axial (C4 level) images.

2. Do the signal abnormalities in these diseases typically begin in the cervical, thoracic, or lumbar region?

3. MR signal abnormalities have been demonstrated in which of the major white matter tracts above the site of a chronic spinal cord injury? Below the injury site?

4. Explain how the postcontrast T1-weighted axial image (C7-T1 level) affects the differential diagnosis.

Wallerian Degeneration

1. Vitamin B_{12} deficiency and vitamin E deficiency.

2. Subacute combined degeneration, secondary to vitamin B_{12} deficiency, usually begins in the thoracic cord.

3. Above—fasciculus gracilis and fasciculus cuneatus (posterior columns). Below—corticospinal tracts.

4. Evidence of surgery for a left foraminal lesion can be seen. Trauma to the posterior surface of the cord or posterior roots at the time of surgery is the most plausible explanation for the wallerian degeneration in the posterior columns.

Reference

Becerra JL, Puckett WR, Hiester ED, et al: MR-pathologic comparisons of Wallerian degeneration in spinal cord injury. *AJNR Am J Neuroradiol* 16:125–133, 1995.

Cross-Reference

Neuroradiology: THE REQUISITES, p 217.

Comment

This 72-year-old woman had a left C8 schwannoma resected 17 years before the imaging study, as well as a long history of loss of proprioception in the lower extremities, left more than the right. The sagittal image demonstrates evidence of laminectomies at C6 and C7, and the axial postcontrast T1-weighted image confirms the C7 laminectomy. Furthermore, this axial image shows enhancement in the left neural foramen, most likely representing postoperative scar plus epidural veins. The T2*-weighted axial image at C4 and the sagittal image clearly show increased signal intensity in the posterior columns above the laminectomy site. The signal abnormality extends to the C2-3 level and is consistent with wallerian degeneration in the posterior columns (ascending white matter tracts).

Wallerian degeneration refers to antegrade degeneration of axons and their accompanying myelin sheaths and results from injury to the proximal portion of the axon or its cell body. The MR imaging manifestations and temporal course of wallerian degeneration that occur above and below a spinal cord injury have been described by Becerra and colleagues in a study comparing MR imaging and histologic results from formalin-fixed postmortem human cords (N = 24). The MR images showed increased signal intensity in the posterior columns above the injury level, as well as in the lateral corticospinal tracts below the injury level, in all cases in which cord injury had occurred 7 or more weeks before death. Injuries occurring 8 to 12 days before death showed no abnormal signal above or below the level, although early wallerian degeneration was present histologically. Thus, in the injured spinal cord, wallerian degeneration is unlikely to be detected between 8 days and 7 weeks postinjury, yet it should become apparent at intervals greater than 7 weeks postinjury. Interestingly, the injured cords did not show the low signal intensity that has been observed on T2-weighted images of cerebral white matter in vivo 4 to 14 weeks after cerebral infarction. In the brain, wallerian degeneration produces hyperintense white matter signal at intervals longer than 14 weeks postinjury.

Notes